MONTEFIORE

MONTEFIORE

The Hospital as Social Instrument,

1884–1984

DOROTHY LEVENSON

Farrar, Straus & Giroux

NEW YORK

Library of Congress Cataloging in Publication Data
Levenson, Dorothy.
   Montefiore: the hospital as social instrument,
1884–1984.
   Includes index.
   1. Montefiore Hospital and Medical Center—History
2. Hospital and community—New York (N.Y.)—History.
3. Bronx (New York, N.Y.)—History. I. Title.
[DNLM: 1. Hospitals, General—History—New York City.
2. Hospitals, Teaching—History—New York City. WX 28
AN7M74L]
RA982.N5M745   1984   362.1'1'09747275   84–6059

ACKNOWLEDGMENTS

I cannot adequately thank all the hundreds of people who helped me with this book: the patients, the doctors, the nurses, the technicians, the hospital workers, and the administrators who talked openly with me and allowed me to watch them at work. I am indebted also to many of them for finding the written and pictorial materials on which this work is based. No consistent effort was made over the years to collect the records at Montefiore. When this project was announced, many people came to me with old volumes that they had rescued from the "flood in the Schiff basement" or that they had found in dusty corners. A letter to the members of the Staff and Alumni Association brought many responses of personal photographs and shared reminiscences, and the Association itself provided seed money for early support.

Two Presidents, Drs. Martin Cherkasky and Carl Eisdorfer, were most supportive of my efforts, as were the two Chairmen of the Board of Trustees during the same years, Robert Tishman and Lawrence Buttenweiser. I was fortunate enough to spend many hours in interviews with Dr. E. M. Bluestone before his death. Many people have read sections of the book, and made suggestions about style and content. While I take responsibility for all matters of judgment or fact, the entire manuscript has been read and criticized by a committee of people most knowledgeable about the history of Montefiore: Edmund Rosenthal, former Chairman of the Board of Trustees; and Drs. Louis Leiter, George Silver, and Harry Zimmerman. My special thanks to them. My thanks also to Irving Gottsegen, who introduced me to Montefiore.

CONTENTS

MONTEFIORE

The Hospital and
Its History

The men who planned the opening of the Montefiore Home for Chronic Invalids in 1884 were philanthropists, not doctors. They wanted to do something for the sick people whom the hospitals of the day could not help: patients with cancer and tuberculosis and syphilis and "the opium habit" and arthritis and chronic kidney disease and chronic melancholy, those for whom there was little hope and no expectation of cure. The medical care provided for these "incurables" was only one form of aid: clean, warm accommodations, careful nursing, good food, and provision for the families of the sufferers were equally important in comforting the dying or bringing them back to some level of functioning.

The first patients filled twenty-six beds in a small frame house on Manhattan's Upper East Side. The modern Montefiore Medical Center sprawls across the unlovely reaches of the northern Bronx, New York City's least glamorous borough, providing care for more than two thousand inpatients in more than forty buildings, and through a network of affiliations and connections that includes the Albert Einstein College of Medicine and frequently leads to accusations of imperial ambition.

Hospitals are the most expensive, intricate, and valued institutions in our society, temples without whose protective presence no community feels safe. As a great teaching hospital, Montefiore is a delicate, complex, paradoxical instrument, functionally dependent on the conscientious performance of repetitive tasks and the brilliance of decisions made in the storm of crisis. At a time when there is no way to measure the geometrically increasing store of scientific knowledge available for use in the care and cure of the sick, these tasks and these decisions are accomplished by people at the lowest and highest extremes of comprehension of that knowledge. Hospitals are equally dependent on the skills of the most honored and rewarded class of professionals in our nation and on the kind of work that many societies, including our own until recently, tend to delegate to their most despised castes. A high level of patient care is sustained equally by the cold eye of scientific detachment and by warm hands ready to comfort all the remembered fears of helpless childhood, by the information that came from the research laboratory this morning, and by those patterns of mutual caring imprinted in the long eons of learning to be human. Hospital management requires above all the ability to persuade a great variety of people to use their skills of heart and mind with an attitude of profound concern for the lives of strangers.

Modern medicine is a child of the scientific-technological revolution but the machines have not replaced the people. They have increased the need for technologists. There are no long wards of sleeping patients watched over by a single nurse with a quiet lamp. In a teaching hospital that does more open-heart operations than appendectomies every year, there are ever-increasing numbers of intensive-care beds, with patients hooked up to machines that must be closely monitored by people educated enough to read the messages sent out by the machines, and the educated are expensive. The cost of technology is not only in the one-time buying of a machine but in the ongoing salaries of the keepers of the machines.

Society relies on teaching hospitals for the delivery of the best of today's medical care, for the transmission of the ability to deliver future care, and for the assurance that tomorrow's care will be better than today's. The education of physicians is firmly based on practical experience in hospitals. The procedures by which the results of research become part of practice take place, to an overwhelming degree, in hospitals. The natural tendency to use existing institutions, instead of inventing new ones, means that most of the recent developments in the delivery of health care, whether accidental or planned, have been linked in one way or another with hospitals.

1

A Confederate Surgeon
Comes North

The founding fathers of Montefiore were men accustomed to change. Most were immigrants, born in Germany. They had the skills to achieve success in a new world. Many of them also found adventure.

Simon Baruch, the first chief of the medical staff, was one of the adventurers. He was a man with an enthusiasm for losing causes. In his youth he followed Lee to Gettysburg. He bound up the wounds of the Southerners who made one last stand against William Tecumseh Sherman. As an old man, he continued to preach the gospel of hydrotherapy, of water as a cure-all, long after medical science passed him by. At times his enthusiasms led him to espouse contradictory causes. He was simultaneously president of the Hebrew Benevolent Association of Camden, South Carolina, and a fervent member of the Ku Klux Klan.

Born in Schwersenz, Prussia, on July 29, 1840, to a father who claimed descent from Baruch the Scribe, editor of the prophecies of Jeremiah, Simon became a student in the Royal Gymnasium at Posen but, at the age of fifteen, fled to the United

States to escape conscription into the Prussian Army. The boy went to live with his mother's sister and her shopkeeper husband in Camden. By day he kept the store's books; at night he learned English, reading American history with a dictionary beside him.

Simon's aunt persuaded her husband to send him first to the South Carolina Medical College in Charleston and then to the Medical College of Virginia in Richmond. While Simon studied anatomy, the Civil War broke out and in April 1862 he joined the Third Battalion, South Carolina Infantry.

The new medical graduate was appointed Assistant Surgeon "without ever having lanced a boil," according to his own account. His first battle experience was at Second Manassas (Second Bull Run by Northern reckoning). The chief business of Civil War surgeons was the removal of wounded limbs. The fear of infection was ever present but there was no widespread understanding of its cause or the ability to cure it. Swift amputation of the arm or leg was seen as a preventive measure.

The young Dr. Baruch also served on the bloody battlefields of Antietam and Gettysburg. (At both sites he was captured by Union troops, but since it was the policy of both the Union and the Confederacy to exchange captured surgeons, he was released each time.) He last saw action in March 1865 in Thomasville, North Carolina, as the Confederacy was making its last stand.

After the surrender Simon went back home to Camden. He married the girl who, according to family legend, saved his portrait from Yankee marauders, fathered children (including that Bernard who was to become the friend and adviser of Presidents), and settled down to the life of a country doctor interested in scientific farming.

The political and economic turmoil of postwar South Carolina curtailed his dream of peace. Cities and farms lay in ruins. The slaves were free but landless and penniless, while their late owners' capital investment had disappeared. The South found in the ex-slave a scapegoat for the anger aroused by inflation, bankruptcy, and social disruption. The Jew who had fled from

Prussia joined his neighbors in the Klan, adopting the whole mythology of the white South, and riding in the bloody campaign in which Wade Hampton and his Redshirts took over the government of South Carolina in 1876.

The end of the Yankee occupation did not bring peace. Violence and poverty continued to torment the South. After the death of a family friend in a duel, the doctor began to consider another emigration. The Baruchs became one of the many Jewish families who moved North as the white Protestant majority drew the line more and more clearly between themselves and all other Southerners. Although he was appointed chairman of the South Carolina Board of Health in 1880, the next year Dr. Baruch sold his farm and practice for a total of $18,000 and took his wife and four sons to New York City.

There, a prosperous Jewish middle class was establishing the network of charitable institutions which in the next twenty years was to expand rapidly to cope with the needs of the flood tide of Eastern European immigration and to provide career opportunities for a growing group of Jewish professionals.

The growing city of New York was one of sharp social contrasts. The rich, untrammeled by income taxes, lived in marble-halled splendor. The poor, unprotected by any system of welfare grants or social security, lived in dirt and poverty, downtown in rat-ridden tenements or uptown in makeshift shanties on the borders of Central Park or the banks of the Hudson River. In sickness or in health, they could look for relief only to the charity of the rich.

In the first weeks the doctor was so worried about making a living in this strange city that he developed psychosomatic symptoms of heart disease. The trouble disappeared when he began to prosper, his reputation growing when he made one of the first diagnoses of appendicitis and recommended surgery over the misgivings of other doctors. He met the men who were planning to set up the Montefiore Home for Chronic Invalids, remaining involved with the Home in one way or another for the next twenty-six years. At the same time he built up a private practice, treated patients at other institutions, taught, and helped found several professional organizations concerned with issues of public health. New York's primitive sanitation system led him to describe Manhattan Island as a "body of land surrounded by sewage" and to successfully advocate the establishment of public baths.

The faucet replaced the knife as his favorite weapon against disease as he became a fervent advocate of hydrotherapy, the use of water applied both externally and internally.

American medical practitioners were not yet agreed upon a body of scientific knowledge as the basis of their craft. The commonly used drugs were frequently ineffective and often dangerous in themselves, purges and opiates prescribed in massive doses for major and minor complaints. Water as a cure-all had long flourished at great European spas.

Medicine was in a time of transition. The information and intuitions which became the foundation of the twentieth century revolution in medicine and health were being collected, but Simon Baruch, in his contradictory beliefs, was typical of the well-informed, conscientious physician of his day. He knew his surgical instruments should be clean. He also believed that water could cure almost anything. The United States, lacking regulations concerning professional education or licensing, had hundreds of doctors who were ignorant, uneducated charlatans. At the same time, brilliant medical research was in progress at the best European universities. Medical practice on both sides of the Atlantic covered the spectrum from the level of that research to medieval superstition.

Medicine was waking from ages-long impotence, but the magic bullets that were to slay the pestilential diseases still terrorizing whole populations were in the future. Infection was the chief cause of death, whether through the sudden fatal fevers of childhood, the slow-moving seeds of tuberculosis or syphilis that took years to kill, the epidemics of cholera and typhoid that regularly swept through the crowded cities, or the bacteria that lurked in operating room or childbed seeking entry to a human host.

In 1879, when he spoke before the Paris Academy of Medicine, Louis Pasteur drew on the blackboard the chains of streptococci that the unbelieving physicians carried on their grubby hands. In 1882, Robert Koch identified the bacillus that caused tuberculosis. In spite of Koch's discovery, tuberculosis was to remain the great plague that decimated the young adults of Europe and North America.

Besides identification of particular microorganisms as the agents of particular diseases, other pieces of information were falling into place. In the early eighties, Admiral Takaki eradicated beriberi from the Japanese Navy by adding milk and meat to the sailors' normal diet of fish and rice.

The knowledge of the causes of infection and the elements of nutrition ultimately fit into a general theory of the functioning of human physiology. Before his death in 1878, Claude Bernard described the *milieu intérieur,* that chemical balance of the fluids within the body which "is the primary condition for freedom and the independence of existence." A recognition of the value of cleanliness, aseptic and antiseptic techniques, and the development of anesthesia allowed surgeons to make dramatic progress. The industrial revolution in the United States and Europe had passed from early concentration on the mechanics of power and was developing the chemistry-based technology that was to interact closely with the progress of medicine.

By the end of the nineteenth century, scientists from many different disciplines knew infinitely more about the human body than was known at the beginning of the period. There had not occurred a corresponding breakthrough in the ability to cure most diseases. There was little that the practicing physician could offer a patient in the way of effective treatment, and the hospitals in which the science and technology were to be used in the future were only slowly taking shape, still performing a quite limited role in society.

Members of the middle class rarely went into a hospital. Big houses, cheap servants, and a surplus of unmarried and unemployed female relatives made accommodation at home possible, with nursing the sick one of the expected domestic skills. The doctor carried a little black bag containing the few drugs he had available. Operations were still often performed on the kitchen table.

The people who went to hospitals were usually those who had no homes or whose homes could not cope with the added burden of nursing an invalid. Most women in maternity hospitals were prostitutes or girls who had committed the ultimate Victorian sin of pregnancy outside marriage. Throughout the nineteenth century male patients outnumbered female patients in New York's general hospitals. Men in any society are more likely to live alone than women, and in a city with a constant stream of arriving immigrants, there was always a large population of unattached males.

The almshouse was an all-purpose institution—part old-age home, part insane asylum, part hospital. All the people who could not function as members of society and had no families able or willing to care for them were there. Almshouses were supported from local taxes. Resistance to spending any unnecessary money was compounded by America's terrible Calvinist suspicion that being poor was a sin.

In part the voluntary hospitals run by volunteer boards of philanthropists were a reaction to the stigma of the almshouse. Hospitals in New York were built to take care of the "deserving poor" so that they would not have to mix with those reduced to poverty and sickness by alcoholism or prostitution or general moral depravity.

Hospitals played little part in the lives of most doctors, who visited and treated their patients at home, where they were nursed by their families, not exposed to the dangers of infection that existed in every hospital. Many doctors trained as apprentices to practicing doctors and did not spend time in hospitals even as students or interns. The hospital was important only to the most advanced medical teaching and research. Consistent observation and comparison of patients was possible under hospital conditions. Education could best be carried out in a hospital, where students and teacher could gather at the bedsides of interesting cases, and since most of those cases were poor people, ill educated, dependent on charity and therefore unlikely to ask questions, new treatments could be tried more easily in hospitals, studies done, papers written. Thus, hospitals were important to a small proportion of the people who became sick and important to a small but influential proportion of the doctors practicing medicine in the United States.

Philanthropy was a much bigger business than medicine in the nineteenth century, as there were almost no publicly supported methods of dealing with the poor, the helpless, the halt, the lame, or the blind. Charity was a duty for those who had some of the goods of this world. There was individual charity and there was a network of orphanages, schools, houses for fallen women, and hospitals. The Montefiore Home for Chronic Invalids was to be a part of this grid, to take care of the people for whom the acute-care hospitals such as Mount Sinai could do no more. As were most charitable institutions, the Home was linked to a particular religious group. Religion formed the organizational frame for philanthropic activity.

Simon Baruch had much in common with the men who established the Home. Most were born in Germany, and many had lived in the South and aided the Confederate cause in one way or another. They banded together in concern for Jewish communal needs, their religious beliefs usually Reform, often agnostic.

There was little anti-Semitism compared to what was to come as the number of Jews in the United States increased. New England theology had always emphasized the Old Testament. There was a certain interest in and respect for God's Chosen People and the religion from which Christianity had sprung.

Some German Jews arrived, like Simon Baruch, with education and family connections, often with enough money to start in business, retaining close ties with their families in Germany, traveling back to visit or to marry. They felt closer to their fellow Teutonic immigrants and to their fellow Americans than they did to the Eastern European Jews, fleeing poverty and pogrom, who were crowding into the tenements of the Lower East Side. These newcomers were often penniless, with little secular education, speaking Russian or Polish or a Yiddish that sounded to German Jews like a barbaric and mutilated form of German. Their clothes were strange, their religion Orthodox, often mystical, their politics frequently revolutionary.

There was another Jewish group in New York City, the Sephardim, descendants of the Jews expelled from Spain and Portugal by Ferdinand and Isabella. The original Sephardic settlers, grudgingly allowed by Peter Stuyvesant to settle in Manhattan, had been penniless. Through the generations, their descendants had gained wealth, security, and a tendency to look upon the brash German newcomers as a threat to their own positions of power.

The Montefiore Home for Chronic Invalids was born of a reasonably simple impulse, to honor the one hundredth birthday of an ex-sheriff of London by doing something for the poor of New York City. Sir Moses Montefiore was the most widely known Jewish leader and philanthropist of the nineteenth century. Born in Italy, he spent most of his life in Great Britain, marrying the sister-in-law of a Rothschild, achieving great wealth, becoming sheriff of London, kneeling before Queen Victoria for a knighthood, using his money and influence to protect his fellow Jews from the depredations of the rulers of the Ottoman and Russian empires. Celebrations of his centennial birthday were worldwide. The schoolchildren of Ramsgate, where he spent his later years, marched singing to his house. The Queen, remote in lifelong mourning for her beloved Albert, sent greetings. In Palestine and in Australia, orphanages and hospitals were named and renamed in his honor. In New York City, the clerk and president of the Congregation of Shearith Israel, the most important Sephardic synagogue in the city, sent out invitations to a meeting to discuss "taking steps to becomingly mark the approaching anniversary."

The men who gathered in the synagogue vestry room on 19th Street on February 4, 1884, were some of the most distinguished members of the New York Jewish community, German and Sephardic. There were nine rabbis, the presidents of Temple Emanu-El and of the United Hebrew Charities, as well as the presidents of the boards of Mount Sinai Hospital, founded before the Civil War, and of the Hebrew Free School Association, trustees of orphan asylums and of relief societies. All were well-to-do men who felt a strong sense of obligation to those less fortunate, well aware of the appalling distance by which they were separated from poorer New Yorkers.

Alexander II of Russia was assassinated in March 1881 and the bomb that killed a Tsar set off one of the great population movements of all time. The pogroms that followed the royal death were to propel more than a million people from the crowded shtetls of Russia and Poland to the noisome tenements and noisy classrooms of Manhattan. Violence and poverty uprooted masses of people everywhere. From 1870 to 1895, more than ten million immigrants arrived in the United States. Many of them landed in New York—and stayed.

The new immigrants changed the country, changed the big cities, and metamorphosed the Jewish community of New York City, which increased from 80,000 to 1,100,000 in thirty years. Most of the newcomers were from Eastern Europe, ragged refugees. Numerically and culturally, they were to overwhelm the German and Sephardic communities.

Jacob Schiff, who had left his own comfortable middle-class family in Frankfurt am Main to found one of the largest fortunes in the United States, pointed out to the philanthropists in the vestry that "there exists in the lower part of our city, a population of Hebrews, which socially stands as low and is no better than those of our race in Eastern Europe, Africa and Asia." He suggested doing something about the terrible housing in which the immigrants lived, perhaps build a "new quarter of improved tenement houses" to be called the Montefiore Tenements.

Mr. M. W. Platzek spoke on behalf of the downtown branch of the Young Men's Hebrew Association and its "Russian mission," which was busy "civilizing and Americanizing the uncouth refugees from barbarity and oppression." A Home for Incurables was proposed by Mr. Adolphus S. Solomons, a visitor from Washington. The rabbis were concerned about juvenile delinquency, and they wanted to set up a reformatory for young

Jewish criminals. The director of the Society for the Prevention of Cruelty to Children liked the idea of the reformatory, as did Mr. Meyer Stern, who considered spending money on the young and healthy a sensible idea. He said that "those who had a lifetime before them should rather be the first recipients of a practical benevolence than those who awaited hopelessly the final dissolution."

Ex-Judge Isaacs worried that a reformatory "was not a graceful tribute to link with Montefiore's name." He preferred something educational, such as the Cooper Institute. Mr. Lewis May agreed. A reformatory was not really necessary since "Mrs. M. D. Lewis, with her tenement visits and dragging the children to school and to refinement, did the work of a dozen reformatories and did it well." The discussion was tense and the meeting adjourned late after the appointment of a committee to consider the plans put forward and to report back in three weeks.

These were men of strong opinions. While the committee deliberated, a four-page printed circular—signed "Justice"—was distributed around the Jewish community. "Justice" was indignant at the very notion of a reformatory, feeling that, in the first place, there were not many young Jews in trouble. "Seldom, very seldom does it happen that a poor Jewish peddler or bootblack boy is brought to the court." These delinquents—few as they are—were frightened at the idea of being placed in a "Catholic or other reformatory." But, said "Justice," "let them once become aware that even if they are convicted of misdemeanor, they will be cared for by Jews and among Jews, and they will consider it a boon to exchange their unpleasant homes at the tenement houses for the comparatively more pleasant ones at the reformatory."

The uproar created by "Justice" had its effect. At the next meeting, on March 7, the rabbis acknowledged that the plan for a reformatory was dead. They threw their weight behind the Home for Incurables. The committee had previously given approval to the home. Mr. Isaac Wallach, vice-president of the board of Mount Sinai Hospital, submitted a "carefully tabulated" report on behalf of the committee stating that fifty invalids could be cared for at a cost of $20,000 a year.

There was a suggestion that the money—yet to be raised—should be placed at the disposal of the managers of Mount Sinai Hospital so that they could say "how it might best be employed," but by the end of the evening another committee had been appointed "to mature plans for the founding of a 'Home for Incurables.' " Five of the members of the committee, including Jacob Schiff and H. S. Allen, who was president, were also trustees of Mount Sinai Hospital, two were from the United Hebrew Charities, and two were trustees of the Home for Aged and Infirm Hebrews. There were two rabbis and four other members.

The decision in favor of the establishment of an institution for the delivery of medical care was in step with the times. During the decade 1880 to 1890, four publicly owned hospitals were founded in New York City, and thirty-two under private and charitable auspices, a reflection of the growth in medical capabilities taking place. Many of them were like Montefiore in that they were planned to take care of special classes of people: Babies' Hospital, Brooklyn Home for Consumptives, Memorial Hospital for the Treatment of Cancer and Allied Diseases, Yorkville Dispensary and Hospital for Women and Children.

One of the first acts of the committee was to send out an appeal for funds with an explanation of the need for a Home for Chronic Invalids (a less terrifying name than the original): "The last annual report of the United Hebrew Charities states that the Institution had to provide partial relief for 174 chronic invalids though the object of the particular charity is to afford relief to the poor, the helpless and transient destitute. . . . Mount Sinai Hospital cannot furnish accommodations for this class of invalids, the beds therein being necessarily required for the large number of patients suffering with acute diseases, who can be benefited by medical treatment, and the Managers of Mount Sinai Hospital are, in consequence, compelled to constantly refuse admission to those afflicted with incurable disease." The proposed home was seen as "a most necessary link in the grand chain of Hebrew Charities which are so noble an ornament of New York Judaism."

The committee wrote to likely supporters with a return-addressed postcard on which the recipient could indicate the amount of support he or she could pledge to the Home—$10 a year for members and $25 a year for patrons. The Home for Chronic Invalids was to be run by a society. Anybody who wanted to become a member submitted his or her name to the Board of Trustees or the Executive Committee for election by the majority. Since membership dues were seen as the financial base of the institution, there was active recruiting and by the end of the first year there were 750 members and 170 patrons.

A life membership cost $250. Larger contributions provided special dividends: $1,000 bought "the privilege of a bed and a room bearing the name of the donor, which may be occupied during the lifetime of such a donor by such person or persons as he may designate, subject to the rules and regulations of the Home"; $2,500 extended the honor of selecting the patient not only to the donor but also to his heirs.

The affairs of the society were to be managed by a board of twelve Trustees, elected by the general membership, fifty persons counting as a quorum.

With no time to build anything very imposing before Sir Moses' birthday in October, the Trustees rented a gaslit frame house on the northeast corner of 84th Street and Avenue A. A neat picket fence ran all the way around the three-story clapboard building. A visitor came from the unpaved street through a gate and up wide steps to a broad veranda that stretched across the front of the house and shaded the lower rooms with their long french windows. Awnings and shutters protected the windows of the two upper stories.

The lease ran for four years, and before the official opening three months were spent making necessary alterations. On the first floor, there was a parlor where an elaborately decorated "Book of Life," in which the names of all contributors were entered, sat on a stand. On the same floor, there was a seven-bed ward for male patients, a female ward with three beds, and a "drugstore."

On the second floor, three rooms became female wards, each with three beds. There was a room each for the matron and the head nurse and two bathrooms, one for each sex. On the top floor there were two more male wards, each with three beds, a large room for servants, a room where the clerk and male nurses slept, and a tiny room for another servant.

The first patient, admitted on October 19, a few days before the official opening, was Louis Spanier, a thirty-year-old painter, born in the United States and then living at 103 First Avenue. Five years before, he had been diagnosed as suffering from "painter's colic"—lead poisoning—and had spent three months in St. Vincent's Hospital. Even before that he suffered from chills and fever every summer, and in 1881 had hemorrhaged from the lungs, losing a "washbasinful of blood." At intervals of about a year he had the same kind of hemorrhage and came to Montefiore, where he was diagnosed as suffering from tuberculosis.

On October 26, 1884, birthday celebrations for Sir Moses were held all over the city. The *World* reported: "In all the synagogues throughout the city the Hebrews celebrated the one hundredth birthday of their noble leader in benevolence. . . . Even the humble congregations on the east side, in their narrow places of worship, had some sprigs of green to twine about the portrait of the great benefactor so dear to them. In the magnificent temples of the wealthy Israelites the floral decorations were more elaborate, but in all the same service, arranged by Rabbi Adler, of London, was read. The text, in Hebrew and English, was furnished to all. The orthodox Hebrews followed the former, while the more reformed brethren used their native languages."

Temple Emanu-El was crowded. Three quarters of the people who came had to be turned away. The principal eulogy was spoken by Henry Ward Beecher (the most popular Christian preacher in New York, able to ask for and get $1,000 as a lecture fee), the brother of Harriet Beecher Stowe, the author of *Uncle Tom's Cabin.*

The Montefiore Home for Chronic Invalids was dedicated on the morning of the twenty-sixth. Henry Allen, the President, welcomed the guests but he was not feeling well. (He was to be succeeded by Jacob Schiff within the year.) Mr. A. L. Sanger read Mr. Allen's address. There were prayers and psalms and more speeches. A memorial tablet was unveiled and a cablegram sent to Sir Moses: "New York makes scheochona [celebration] over opening of Montefiore Home for Chronic Invalids, with imposing ceremonies today. Our congratulations to you."

Sir Moses was not to live long after the great birthday. He died on July 28, 1885, six days after the death of Ulysses S. Grant. In public addresses, the names of the two heroes were linked with the pious hope that they "would doubtlessly meet at the footstool of the merciful God of all."

An engraving of Sir Moses was put on display in the parlor, black draperies were hung, and the patients said Kaddish (the prayer for the dead) for a month.

The Home was already fulfilling its purposes as defined in the bylaws: "To afford permanent shelter in sickness and to relieve invalids residents [sic] of the City of New York belonging to the Hebrew faith, who by reason of the incurable character of the disease from which they may be suffering are unable to procure permanent medical treatment in any of the Hospitals or Homes."

That seemed simple enough, but in practice the Trustees struggled hard over many years, refining and redefining their goals, for, as they said in their first annual report, "the responsibility of the Executive Committee was both novel and embarrassing, for as they were not aware of the existence of any similar charity based exclusively upon the admission of non-paying beneficiaries, rules and regulations had to be established, and from time to time changes made, based upon the results of actual experience."

At the annual meeting in 1887 Mr. Wallach offered an amendment which removed the words "belonging to the Hebrew faith" from the bylaws and thus made the Home nonsectarian. The amendment was accepted with the promise that "all religious ceremonies practiced in the Home must be in accordance with the Jewish faith. This shall not, however, preclude the attendance of a clergyman of any other faith at the solicitation of a patient."

The Home was to be managed not by the professional staff but by the Executive Committee of the Board of Trustees: "To the Executive Committee shall be confided a general superintendency of the Home. They shall make rules and regulations for their government subject to the approval of the Board. They shall have the power to accept or reject applications for admission to the Home, purchase all articles required for its use, and keep a faithful record of their proceedings. Three or more of their number to form a Visiting Committee. It shall be the duty of the Visiting Committee to inspect the Home weekly, if possible, and notice any dereliction of duty on the part of the employees, to see that the wards are kept in a cleanly condition, examine the food and the manner in which it is prepared for the use of the patients, and generally to make such suggestions for the improvement of the Institution as in their judgment they may deem necessary."

The first year was a financial success. Income, none of it from patients, was almost twice expenditures. Receipts totaled $34,184.44. Dues from patrons, members, and life members added up to $15,080. The balance was made up of donations ranging from $2,500 each from Jacob Schiff and Louis Gans to 50 cents from one, L. Bauman.

The donations of articles that year had a homely simplicity. Mrs. E. J. King gave three pairs of rubbers, one pair of boots, three pairs of slippers, one pair of shoes, six suits of clothing, seven smoking gowns, two sets of underwear, one dozen handkerchiefs, seven nightcaps, one silk cap, one cane, four pairs of eyeglasses, one invalid chair, one pair of crutches, and one pair of gloves. All gifts, however small, were listed in the annual report. Mrs. Straus gave one glass of jelly, and S. H. Bleier supplied two tarts. Strawberries and ice cream were donated as treats for the patients. Concern for appropriate arrangements for the dead was reflected in the gift of a velvet funeral pall. (The Trustees did not believe that their duty to a patient ended at the time of death. A piece of ground was given for a cemetery by Congregation Beth El. In the second year of operation $278.33 was spent on funerals for deceased patients.)

The Young Ladies' Sewing Society was soon at work and in one year produced forty-six nightgowns, eight flannel night-sacks, eight calico nightsacks, fifty-eight towels, thirteen aprons, ten skirts, two suits, sixteen chemises, forty-one pillowcases and thirty-six handkerchiefs.

To increase the flow of donations from the public, the Trustees resorted to the flowery excesses of Victorian prose style: "Beginning with less than half a dozen patients, there had not been a period during the past year when the limited capacity of the Home has not made it painfully necessary to refuse admission to many worthy applicants, who in most cases returned to their poverty stricken homes, suffering disappointment, made doubly sensitive by aggravated pain, and with prayer on their parched and quivering lips, to hasten the blessed time when the further liberality of the dear, good friends of the Home will enable its Directors to extend the area of its ministrations commensurate with the constantly increasing demands upon its bounty."

The plight of rejected applicants provoked more than purple prose. The Trustees decided: "To measurably help the most worthy unsatisfied claimants, . . . to care in part for a limited number of them at their homes, by allowances of a small sum of money every month, and the personal attention, as far as his time will permit, of our Resident Physician."

The minutes of the Executive Committee show the members' close attention to detail and how much administrative work they did. They handled all admissions and therefore had to struggle with hard decisions about the ultimate purpose of the Home. From the beginning it was decided that "the Committee consider no application for admission into this institution unless it be accompanied by the certificate of the attending physician of a hospital attesting that the applicant is suffering from an incurable disease."

Applicants were rejected for reasons other than the possibility of recovery. Sufferers from Poughkeepsie and Cleveland were unacceptable because they were not residents of New York City. Some were turned down because of age—or because their problems seemed to be those of old age more than specific disease: "M.D., number 23, not a fit case for admission into this institution. He was advised to apply at the Home for the Aged and Infirm." Some cases were more difficult to decide. On September 27, 1885, J.M. was sent to Bellevue Hospital "for examination as to his sanity." On October 4 he was readmitted to Montefiore Home since the doctor at Bellevue felt that he, "though not positively insane, was not to be held accountable for his actions." The little rented house did not have facilities for caring for the insane and that had not been the intention of the founders, but there was a philosophy of finding some kind of help for sufferers wherever possible. Another opinion was sought.

"Dr. Blake, Superintendent of Charities and Corrections of the Outdoor Poor Department [of the City of New York], recommended the Long Island Home Hotel for Nervous Invalids at Amityville, Long Island, as a proper place for the patient."

Mr. M. was consulted, and "having signified a willingness to be removed and to provide for his board and support from the pension received from the government, Doctor Rice [the resident physician] was directed to have him sent to the above institution the following week. In order to help pay his board in advance, in an anticipation of the pension installment that he received, it was resolved to make him a donation of Twenty Dollars."

In 1886, it was decided: "Cases of epilepsy and other diseases especially of a surgical character [i.e., abscesses or infected wounds] which rendered the patients offensive to persons with whom they came into continued contact were not admitted. . . . It has also been necessary to limit, in a measure, the number of cases of pulmonary phthisis [tuberculosis], with which by far the largest proportion of applicants are affected, in order that it may not be necessary to associate them with patients who would be harmed thereby."

Some patients did not take refusal easily. Mrs. B. first applied complaining of rheumatic pains all over her body. The doctor who examined her concluded that she was not sick enough for the Home. The forty-three-year-old Mrs. B. then took poison of a type which burned her esophagus. This gained her admission and treatment for both conditions.

The Trustees were aware from the beginning of the impact of chronic illness upon the lives of patients and their families. They were not dealing with people ill for a period of time and then able to resume their ordinary lives. The Trustees made efforts at long-term rehabilitation. Some patients were helped to start life again in a more suitable climate: "W., a 62-year old tinsmith from Germany, having decided to go to Europe, it was resolved to appropriate the sum of twenty dollars to assist him in making the voyage. C., choosing to go to California, an appropriation not exceeding fifty dollars was voted him." C. later died in California and left $250 to the Home. When seventy-one-year-old C.M. applied to the Home she was admitted "provided the children are cared for." On May 10, 1885, L.M., applying for admission, was reported as "at present under the care of the Society for the Prevention of Cruelty to Children." The fifteen-year-old girl was admitted for "incontinence of urine." In the atmosphere of the Home, probably kinder than that of her previous environment, she improved, but had no home to which to return. Two years later L.M.'s name was moved "from the Patients' list to the servants' list."

Nineteenth-century hospitals often used patients to do the housekeeping and some of the nursing. When almost all patients were poor, many of them, such as L.M., had no families to which to return and were glad to remain at the hospital. The long tradition of patients as workers remained at Montefiore for many years since the needs of the patients for rehabilitation and a role in life long outlasted the need of the institution for cheap, captive labor.

While most patients were admitted purely as charity cases, strong attempts were made to extract payment from relatives where possible. When one patient "had improved materially and . . . it had been discovered that he had wealthy relatives closely connected to him living in the city whose duty it should be to provide for him, it was moved and seconded that Mr. Gans as a

Committee of One call upon the relatives, that he present the case to them and make arrangements for the discharge of the patient." The secretary reported that the board for Mrs. M. had not been paid for two months. "It was therefore moved and carried that the son of Mrs. M. be informed that the patient will be sent home unless her board is paid by Wednesday next." On the next Sunday, "as Mrs. M.'s bill had not been paid up it was resolved to discharge her."

On the other hand, special comforts could be provided by relatives willing to pay for them: "The proposal made by a relative to supply a nurse for the patient was accepted and it was resolved that he be admitted temporarily on condition it was decided to place the patient in a special room."

Patients were allowed to leave the Home for occasional visits with their families. The Executive Committee minutes for March 23, 1889, note "a letter from several patients asking permission to have the privilege of joining their families for Pesach Seder [Passover service] nights. Granted on condition that they return by 11 o'clock." Not everybody came back. P.K., who had TB, "asked permission to go downtown yesterday afternoon. Has not returned. Discharged."

Absences without leave were frowned upon but were sometimes forgiven, as when "the doctor reported that S.R. had been absent from the home for one evening, his absence being caused by temporary insanity, and had returned to the Home with his wife."

The patients were sometimes unruly. A Dr. Daniels wrote to the Executive Committee complaining that a patient had struck a nurse. Mr. Schiff reported that "he had investigated the case and suggested that as the patient had been removed to a separate ward and the nurse was about to leave . . . the matter had been laid over." Mr. Schiff suggested that the following sign be posted in all the wards, written in English, German, and Hebrew: "Officers and nurses must be implicitly obeyed. Complaints can be made to the House Physician or to the Superintendent. Failure to comply with this rule will cause immediate discharge for the offender."

This was no idle threat. Patients were discharged as often for bad behavior as for medical cause. F.G. was twenty-one years old, had tuberculosis, and lied about her bowels, maintaining at one point that she had not had a bowel movement for twelve days, although a rectal examination by a physician did not reveal the mass that such a condition would have produced. She also refused to eat and was finally transferred to Bellevue Hospital for her "disobedience," while another patient, also accused of being "refractory," "promised to do better."

Patients were discharged for infringement of the regulations, regardless of their medical condition, and even when their behavior seemed to be a result of that condition.

In spite of the emphasis on discipline, patients were able to refuse treatments that were classed as "operative procedures." All operations performed required not only the consent of the patient but also that of the Executive Committee of the Board of Trustees. Patients who refused, either permanently or temporarily, to undergo an operation were still kept at the Home and other treatment continued.

In the first months, the day-to-day medical affairs of the Home were under the direction of Dr. Ludwig Senff, the resident physician. The term "resident" implied a doctor who lived on the premises, not the modern meaning of a young doctor in training. Dr. Senff was an experienced man. Born in Schievelbein, Germany, in 1832, he was educated as a doctor at the University of Berlin and then became a military surgeon. He served in three Prussian wars and was awarded the Iron Cross by the Emperor. After the death of his wife, he left his two sons in Berlin and went to London with his two daughters. Leaving the girls in London, he arrived in New York in the middle of 1884 with a letter of introduction to Dr. Froelich, who had been asked to organize the medical staff at the Home, and when the Home opened in October, Dr. Senff was appointed resident physician. His term of office was short. He developed chronic Bright's disease and himself became a patient. As his condition worsened, he was transferred to Mount Sinai Hospital, where he died on January 19, 1885.

Dr. Senff was succeeded by Dr. Joseph M. Rice, who was paid $360 a year, the same amount as Mrs. Fischer, the matron. There were three male nurses, each receiving $15 a month, with one, Solomons, "to be paid $5 extra for mechanical services." The two female nurses were paid at the rate of $12 a month.

Nursing was still a young profession. Nursing schools in the United States were little more than ten years old. Montefiore drew its trained nurses from Mount Sinai. Nineteenth-century sensibilities were offended at the idea of educated young women in operating rooms or caring for male patients. There were battles within many hospitals over the role that nurses were to play. At Montefiore, as in many other institutions, economic considerations won out over the proprieties. In September 1886, Dr. Rice reported: "On August 1, the plan of having female nurses attend the male patients was introduced. . . . I find it a success. Besides being advantageous in the way of nursing, it is a saving of considerable expense as it enables us to diminish the number of employees."

There were problems in the recruiting of attending staff—doctors in private practice who would donate their time to assist the resident physician in caring for the patients. In March the Board of Trustees tartly observed: "Whereas, Dr. Froelich has failed after frequent requests to do so, to organize the medical staff and the medical necessities of the institution require immediate action, it is resolved that a special committee be appointed to select a Chief of Staff in his place."

The next meeting of the Board was set for April 26, but since that was the day of the annual meeting of the trustees of the Hebrew Orphan Asylum, an institution with which many of the members of the Montefiore Board were involved, a special meeting was called for Sunday, April 19, at 10:30 a.m., to ratify the appointment of Dr. Simon Baruch as Chief of Staff.

Dr. Baruch was able to gather a staff of doctors willing to give free care to charity patients. Willy Meyer was consulting surgeon, and Henry S. Oppenheimer, consulting oculist. Three visiting physicians, Emil Hochheimer, Benjamin Morjé, and Charles J. Sharretts, each served four months at a time. The men organized themselves as the "Consulting Board of Physicians," with Dr. Morjé as secretary and Simon Baruch as chairman.

In complying with the request from the Board of Directors "to exercise a general supervision over the medical and hygienic management of the institution," Dr. Baruch visited "from time to time." He found Dr. Rice "conscientious and efficient." From the beginning, the Home was a center of medical education, with thirteen interns spending some time there during the first year.

In June 1885, Dr. Rice threatened to resign but changed his mind after a discussion of his complaints with the Executive Committee. A year later, he left to set up private practice at 3 West 125th Street. Dr. Baruch went carefully through the credentials of the many who applied for the position and finally chose Dr. Charles Schram, who had been house physician at Massachusetts General Hospital.

In philosophical agreement with Baruch, Schram felt that "recovery or permanent improvement cannot be thought of in a large majority of cases. Then, it must be our aim to ameliorate suffering, secure comparative comfort and rescue the unhappy afflicted ones from the gloom of despair."

Alcohol was freely used as a pain-killer and stimulant even by Schram and Baruch, who mistrusted most drugs. A "nutritious diet" for a patient with tuberculosis included: "Beef steaks, eggs. Milk punch every morning and a glass of wine for dinner." This patient remarked that she "sleeps very well after opium." The control of pain was an important part of the therapy, perhaps the most important part for many of the patients, and, besides, alcohol was long thought to have nutritional qualities. Thirty years later, the *Journal of the American Medical Association* was still seriously discussing the maximum dosage of alcohol to provide the greatest food value.

In the second year of operation, the alcoholic supplies included $400.21 worth of wines and brandies bought out of operating funds, plus ten gallons and thirty-six bottles of wine and fifty-three kegs of beer donated by friends of the institution. All this alcohol was divided among the forty-nine patients who were treated in the course of twelve months, thirty-two male and seventeen female. Only five of them gave "United States" as their nationality. Nineteen were from Germany, thirteen were Russian, seven Austrian, four English, and one French. Their occupations were varied. Eleven were "housewives" and two of "no occupation." But the others were cigar makers, clerks, dressmakers, furriers, laborers, merchants, newspaper dealers, pocketbook makers, printers, painters, peddlers, servants, tinsmiths, and truckmen. There was one teacher, one sailor, one "conductor," and one "officer."

While the Board of Directors insisted on proof that the applicant was "incurable" before he or she could be considered for admission, Dr. Baruch pointed with pride to the restoration of some patients, "four to partial usefulness, and three even to health," as the greatest achievement of that first year of work. As long as he was at Montefiore, he continued to argue with the Board about the purposes of the Home. Always in vigorous pursuit of cure or improvement, he had no patience with those who derived emotional satisfaction from "the tender care of the incurable sick."

The work of treating tubercular patients continued: of the twenty-five admitted in 1887, seven died, seven deteriorated rapidly, six remained stable, and five improved their state of health. The symptoms by which their conditions were judged were weight (taken at regular intervals), cough, expectoration, fever, appetite, and night sweats. There is no record of the doctors testing the sputum for the bacillus at Montefiore before 1890.

The doctors relied on their observations of the patient—the general appearance, the cough, the blood or sputum that was brought up, and the sounds they heard coming from the lungs. They struggled to distinguish and find terms for the sounds they heard, the rales and wheezes that told them so much. The problem of differentiating the qualities of sounds in words was troubling—and not really solved until modern electronics made possible wave-form pictures of sounds. As medical students and residents, they spent long hours listening to those mysterious bubblings and crepitations and cracklings that came through their stethoscopes—the best indications of the presence of tuberculosis or bronchitis or emphysema, and the location and extent of damage to the lung—until X-rays provided a glimpse into the dark.

Dr. Schram reported that two new treatments had been tried at Montefiore, without success in either case, although other institutions had apparently found them helpful. The first was the Berjeon method. Sulfurated hydrogen, the gas that smells like rotten eggs and is so beloved by high school chemistry students, was introduced into the bowels using carbonic acid as the vehicle. Five patients suffered this treatment for two months without any improvement. Dr. Schram hastened to assure the Directors that none of the patients "were injured by the treatment, either directly or remotely." He does not mention the attitude of other patients exposed to the smell.

The second experiment was with overfeeding. A rubber tube was introduced into the stomach and through it, after the stomach had been washed out, a predigested meat food was poured in. Three patients bore this for three weeks, but then they complained so much that the treatment had to be abandoned.

A pleasanter experiment was conducted with some patients: "A few of the consumptives, who bear a proportion of fully sixty percent to the other diseases from which our patients suffer, have been sent to elevated geographical regions, in order to test, in a small way and at a slight expense, the desirability of climatic influence upon certain stages and conditions of that fell disease, and with the hope that if valued lives are not positively saved, they may be at least prolonged without acute suffering for many years. At the proper time our medical staff will advise us for proper action in the future."

The standard and preferred treatment for tuberculosis at the Home consisted of three kinds of measures—Hygienic, Medicinal, and Moral (capitalized in the nineteenth-century style). While sufferers from tuberculosis "whose lives are fortified by friends and wealth" often had "constant and exalted hope," Dr.

Schram saw that "it is different at an institution like ours. The continued association with patients exhibiting the distressing symptoms of the disease in its different stages exerts a depressing influence. Under such circumstances it is no easy matter to rekindle the dying embers of hope, rescue the patient from the fatal grasp of despair."

"Hygienic" measures involved fresh air, sunshine, and good food. In summer, Dr. Schram found that the air in the rooms could be kept fresh and at an even temperature. In winter, the inadequate heating and ventilating system made this impossible. Patients, warmly dressed, were encouraged to get as much fresh air as possible at all times of the year.

Food was "plain and nutritious." There were four meals "served during the day, i.e., 7, 12, 3 and 6. In addition, however, nearly all the patients were given a light luncheon at 10 a.m. consisting of milk, cocoa, tea, eggnog, broth or tea and bread. Extras, such as eggs, steaks, chops, chickens, etc., are ordered for those whose appetites are more delicate." The list of "extras" raises questions about the ingredients in the normal meals.

Dr. Schram was attempting to cut down on the use of alcohol. "About a year ago the stronger stimulants were administered freely. These were gradually reduced in amount, and by degrees omitted, so that at present there are but four patients who receive either whiskey or brandy. Wine or beer is given to all. Either sherry or claret, according to the requirements of the case, is employed." Medicinal treatment was twofold in purpose, the first intent being palliative: "All symptoms which tended to debilitate were, as far as possible, relieved. The most distressing of these were loss of appetite, cough, hemorrhage from the lungs, shortness of breath, hectic [the persistent but fluctuating fever typical of tuberculosis] and sleeplessness." The staff was careful of side effects: "In employing drugs for these various purposes, care had also to be taken not to bring upon the patient evils as bad or worse than those from which he or she was to be relieved." Oxygen was administered to patients with intense difficulty in breathing. "Tonic medicines" were used to build up the strength of the patients, especially extract of malt and iron.

"Cod liver oil could be employed with less frequency than might have been desired. It demands a power of assimilation such as few patients possessed." The patients were carefully watched for signs of improvement. "Of the 15 cases, an accurate record of whose weight could be kept, 7 gained, 6 lost, and 2 remained about the same." A variation of half a pound or less was disregarded. Religion occasionally interfered with treatment, as when patients insisted on fasting on Yom Kippur against the advice of doctors.

Dr. Schram was pleased that four patients had improved sufficiently to be discharged. Two men were well enough to earn a living. One was in the Home for two years with "Chronic Catarrh of the stomach"—some kind of digestive problem. The other was in the Home for nine months with "empyema and circumscribed chronic catarrhal pneumonia"—an accumulation of pus in the lungs. In this case, surgical intervention was necessary. A needle or tube was inserted through walls of the chest into the lung to drain off the fluid.

A sixty-four-year-old man admitted with a chronic inflammation of the bladder was intensively treated, catheterized, and his bladder "washed" for nine months, after which he seemed cured and was admitted to the Home for Aged and Infirm Hebrews.

Four patients were in the later stages of syphilis: two men and one woman with tabes dorsalis, and one man with general paresis of the insane. The particular organism that causes syphilis had not yet been discovered. There was no blood test, and no effective treatment.

Syphilis (in its later stages) and tuberculosis were to be important diseases affecting large numbers of patients at Montefiore until the 1950s, when effective treatments were available.

Another disease that has remained central to the operations of the hospital appeared: ". . . a woman about 20 years of age had been suffering with diabetes mellitus for several months. Without being subjected to the restricted diet, usual in such cases, the treatment first adopted by Martineau in 1875, and successfully applied in 67 out of 70 cases, was instituted. After a week, the thirst which is so distressing a feature of this disease, disappeared. At the end of the seven weeks, the patient had apparently returned to her usual state of health. Nor did any physical evidence of her disease remain. Thinking herself permanently cured, she left the Home against advice. As her circumstances were such that she could not continue the same treatment at home, her disease, as had been anticipated, recurred." In spite of the doctor's confidence in Martineau's treatment, it seems likely that the woman's diabetes would have continued to plague her even had she remained in the Home. Her treatment consisted of the elimination of potatoes and wheat bread from her diet and the addition, each day, of a quart of soda water in which an arsenic compound was dissolved.

CHAPTER

2

Men, Women, and Money

Between the Jews of Western Europe, including those who had emigrated to the United States, and the Jews of Eastern Europe, lay a great gap of attitude and experience. The two groups looked at each other in amazement; outsiders saw them as widely separated by dress, manners, mores, politics, language, and religious practice.

Throughout the nineteenth century, a gradual relaxing of anti-Jewish law and anti-Jewish sentiment occurred in many countries west of the Prussian Marches. In England, a Jew, Benjamin Disraeli, became Prime Minister. In Germany, professions and careers opened to Jewish aspirants. So swift was the process of adaptation to the customs of the wider community that Baron Maurice de Hirsch, the German Jewish philanthropist, could agree with Henry Ward Beecher that the problem would be solved by conversion, declaring in an interview in the New York *Times*: "The salvation of the Jews is assimilation, let them be amalgamated by Christianity and merged into Christianity."

The half of the world's Jewish population that was subject to the Tsar had not taken part in this march toward acceptance, living in a land which lagged far behind the rest of Europe in progress toward industrialization or democracy. Confined for hundreds of years to the shabby cities and shtetls—the villages —of the Pale, the sandy plain that was the western border of the Russian Empire, impoverished and persecuted, they were nourished on the slenderest of resources, their own complex culture, grafting onto the stem of the dialect they had brought with them from medieval Germany the branches that were to bear the flowering of the Yiddish language. Their ancient religion developed new forms of learning and mysticism. Impoverished, confined, persecuted, they were given a small measure of relief by Tsar Alexander II; no longer were boys of twelve conscripted and converted; more Jews were allowed to live in cities, to engage in normal business life, to attend school with Russian students. The bomb that cut short Alexander's life ended this glimpse of freedom and replaced it with the reality of terror. The Jewish students were expelled from school. A constantly closing network of regulations concerning business or residence made the making of a living, or even a home, a near-impossibility. The ultimate horror was the official sanction given to pogroms. Raids on Jewish villages, houses, and synagogues, the destruction of homely possessions and religious treasures, the rape of daughters and the beating of sons, had always occurred in the Pale. Now, the government in Moscow, shaken by fears for its own survival under the long shadow of revolution cast by turbulent peasants and theorizing intelligentsia alike, diverted attention from the coming storm by encouraging violence against the shtetls. From 1881 to 1906, the pogrom was official policy. Thousands of Jews were killed and injured, whole districts devastated.

The combination of fear and increasing poverty drove hundreds of thousands of Jews out of Russia. Baron de Hirsch rapidly began spending his fortune to help, including an unsuccessful bribe of one million francs to the Russian government for a promise to allow him to set up technical and agricultural schools for his co-religionists. The Baron shared with many Sephardic and German Jews an almost total lack of knowledge of the background of the people he tried to save, not even being sure what language they spoke. Yiddish, he thought, was "a sort of Hebrew." In spite of his ignorance of the culture he was busy rescuing, the Baron brought thousands of refugees to the United States. Other organizations proffered aid but were overwhelmed by the poverty, by the ill health, and, above all, by the numbers. Forty thousand Eastern European immigrants arrived in New York in 1881 and 1882. Two hundred thousand arrived in the next decade. The Hebrew Emigrant Aid Society despaired: "We as a Society and American citizens cannot and will not be parties to the infliction upon our community of a class of emigrants, whose only destiny is the hospital, the infirmary, or perhaps the workhouse."

The Society, unable to cope, went out of business, to be replaced by the Hebrew Immigrant Aid Society, which had a clearer sense of mission, reflected in the change in title, and survived to welcome generations of refugees.

These Jews fleeing Russia were part of two enormous population movements. Between 1880 and 1924 4 million Jews left Eastern Europe. More than three quarters of them came to the United States as part of an even greater shift of people. The whole continent of Europe was on the move. Industrialization and changing patterns of agriculture upset old ways; railroads and steamships provided quick, cheap transportation. In the century that ended in 1930, 40 million Europeans emigrated to new homes overseas. In the early 1900s, 1.5 million people left Eastern and Southern Europe each year. Most of them came to the United States, and New York was the port of entry for many of them.

The numbers were overwhelming. From 1815 to 1860, 5 million immigrants came to the United States; from 1860 to 1890, 10 million; from 1890 to 1914, 15 million. They came to a country extravagantly rich in natural resources but lacking the social organization to deal with the needs of this flood of people. Apart from a brief inspection at Ellis Island, or a less adequate survey at other ports such as Boston or Baltimore, the immigrants were on their own, often an easy prey for dishonest travel agents, lawyers, and interpreters. Most of the newcomers stayed in the cities.

The Eastern European Jewish immigration was unique in the degree to which the process was assisted and protected by institutions and forms of organization familiar to the people involved. Jewish European and American philanthropic bodies assisted much of the escape from terror. The subsidies were sometimes grudgingly given, often inefficiently administered, often designed to fulfill the dreams of the philanthropist more than those of the emigrant, but many thousands were helped with money and tickets and many more benefited from the network of services set up by the Sephardim and the German Jews. The newcomers might resent the patronizing air with which help was given by those who found their language and their customs strange. They were, however, accustomed to expect and to use the services that were part of their experience of community. In a few years they were able to set up their own hospitals and settlement houses and old-age homes. Jacob Schiff took for granted his obligation to his "fellow Israelites." They, in turn, took for granted his duty to them—and their obligation to each other. Other immigrants often had to painfully learn the uses of the service institutions—the hospitals and schools of a new land. Jewish immigrants expected that their own community would provide help and reacted with pleasure to the fact that so many of the public services of the new country were open to them.

For the United States, this was an era in which capitalism and capitalists flowered, the era of Robber Barons when great fortunes were made in banking and railroading or a combination of both, when there were no antitrust laws to inhibit the acquisition of wealth, no income tax to bite into the wealth acquired, and a public acceptance of the public display of the fruits of wealth.

This was the right time for Jacob Schiff. He came to the United States from Frankfurt am Main, where at one time in the ghetto Judengasse the "ship" sign of the Schiffs and the "red shield" of the Rothschilds hung side by side on the same two-family house. Jacob liked to trace his ancestry back to King Solomon, and while that claim may have had some weak links, he did come from a family long distinguished in scholarship and prosperous in business.

At eighteen, Jacob was in New York and had founded his own brokerage firm before he was old enough to legally sign the partnership papers. Success came to him, however, not as head of his own company. On a trip back to Frankfurt he met Abraham Kuhn, who suggested that he ask Kuhn, Loeb in New York for employment. Schiff found not only a job with a private banking firm second only to J. P. Morgan in the United States but also a bride. The girl he chose to marry, Therese Loeb, had been brought up to subservience and self-effacement by her step-mother. Jacob reassured his family that he had not selected the kind of American girl who was beginning to scandalize the mothers of well-brought-up young European women. He devoted his energies to making his father-in-law's company dominant in railroad financing in the United States.

Schiff went on to make one of the great American fortunes and, as the power and influence of the American Jewish community increased, to rival the worldwide personal charisma that surrounded Sir Moses Montefiore in his lifetime. In 1885 his father-in-law retired and Jacob Schiff became the head of Kuhn, Loeb. That same year, he succeeded Henry Allen as President of the Board of Trustees of the Montefiore Home, a position he held until 1920, the year of his death.

Schiff liked to help adventurous do-gooders. One of the favorites, Lillian Wald, was herself a daughter of the comfortable German Jewish middle class, who grew up in Rochester in upstate New York. After training as a nurse at the New York Hospital's School of Nursing, she planned to study to become a physician. Her background brought her into touch with the Jewish philanthropic establishment, and Betty Loeb, Jacob Schiff's mother-in-law, asked her to teach classes in sanitation and nutrition to immigrant women on the Lower East Side. There, Wald was profoundly moved by the disease, the dirt, and the overcrowding.

Jacob Schiff bought Lillian Wald the house at 265 Henry Street, and her nursing services became the nucleus of the Henry Street Settlement. Wald shared the prejudices of her class toward the objects of her charity: ". . . the more intimately we come to know these poor Russian Jews, the more frequently we are rewarded with unexpected gleams of attractiveness." Some of the patients were sent to Montefiore:

"Annie P., 44 Allen Street, front tenement, second floor. Husband Louis P. came here three years ago and one year ago sent for wife and three children. From that time unfortunately, his trade, that of shoemaker, became less remunerative. She helped by washing and like labor, but two months ago he deserted her, though she stoutly maintains that he returned to Odessa to get his old work back. The youngest, Meyer P., age 5 years, fell from the table and injured his hip. He lay for seven months in the Orthopedic Hospital, 42nd Street; he was discharged as incurable and supplied with a brace. I found them eating, as I have told in the letter to Mr. Schiff. The mother is absolutely tied by her pregnant condition; the cripple is in pain and cries to be carried. . . . Monday I filed application with Montefiore Home for Meyer's admission. As soon as an answer is received from the Montefiore application, I will take the mother to the Nursery and Child's Hospital, where she will be cared for during confinement."

At the dinner which marked his retirement as President of the Board of Trustees of the Montefiore Home in 1920, a speaker referred to the past forty years as the "Schiff era in American Jewry."

The links among members of the Board of Trustees of Montefiore were social, ethnic, religious—and related to business. When the Pennsylvania Railroad wanted to enter New York City and compete with the New York Central, there was opposition from powerful interests in New York and New Jersey. Jacob Schiff called on his friend and fellow Trustee Isidor Straus, whose main interest was the retail trade. By that time, the Straus family controlled two great department stores—Abraham & Straus in Brooklyn and Macy's in Manhattan—and was influential enough in New York business and real estate matters to help Schiff.

The wives of the Board members were also serious and devoted to good works. Like Mrs. Schiff, they were brought up to be as dutiful as wives as they had been as daughters. Mrs. Straus achieved fame by refusing to desert Isidor on the deck of the *Titanic*.

As German-American Jewish women, they were the products of three societies, each with its own rigid rules about the role of women. Well-brought-up European women were heavily chaperoned before marriage and hemmed in by strict rules of decorum afterwards. American women were allowed more social freedom, but almost as few legal rights.

Marriage, usually arranged by the families, and motherhood, were the goals for which women were trained. As immigrants, however, they were expected to appear subservient while they led lives that called for physical and emotional strength, were expected to go through the same hardships as their husbands, scrimping and saving in the lean years, learning a new language and new ways, testing religious and moral beliefs in a new society, and bearing children in pain and danger, far from the comfort of familiar faces and friendly customs.

Their religion and their community encouraged intense involvement in philanthropy, which provided an outlet for their intelligence and their energy. The wives and daughters took as active and creative a role as the husbands and fathers in designing the institutions that were to serve their community's needs in a society struggling with the overwhelming tides of urbanization and immigration, although they were not to achieve seats on the Montefiore Board of Trustees for fifty years.

Mrs. Simon Baruch followed this approved model of domesticity. When her son Bernard started at City College, Mrs. Baruch made over his father's coats for him to wear. Bernard was already close enough to his ultimate six feet three inches to make the wearing of his father's pants impractical.

Much of the social life of the well-to-do Jewish community revolved around philanthropy. Balls, fairs, and plays were organized to raise money for good causes and to allow the marriageable young to meet under the watchful eyes of parents. The first money-raising entertainment for the Montefiore Home was a performance of *Iolanthe* given by the Ladies' Dramatic Union on March 29, 1884, with "Superb Costumes, Special Scenery, Souvenirs," which raised $1,467.10. The Honorary Managers included Grover Cleveland, Carl Schurz, Roscoe Conkling, and Andrew Carnegie as well as such prominent Jewish women as Mrs. Jacob Schiff, Mrs. Jesse Seligman, and Emma Lazarus.

Next year came two great social and financial successes. The Annual Charity Ball under the management of the Purim Association was given at the Metropolitan Opera House for the benefit of the Montefiore Home and brought in $10,255. This ball was an annual event from 1866 to 1902. The Association was made up of young men of the best German Jewish families and raised money for such good causes as the Young Men's and Young Women's Hebrew Associations, the United Hebrew Charities, the Hebrew Orphan Asylum, the Emma Lazarus Downtown Club, and the Russian Emigrant Fund. As many as 3,000 revelers attended, dressed as such Purim-related characters as Queen Esther or Mordecai or such non-Jewish persons as Louis XIV, Queen Isabella, Mother Goose, Charles I, or Pocahontas.

By May 1886, the Trustees had purchased the land for a new Home "on the Boulevard [Broadway] bounded by 138th and 139th Streets." They planned to erect a "plain, substantial building . . . capable of sheltering at least 75 patients." To raise the necessary money, a "Grand Fair" was planned, to run from December 6 to December 18, again under the auspices of the Purim Association, at the New Central Park Garden on the corner of Eighth Avenue and 59th Street.

Months of preparation culminated in the raising (after expenses were paid) of $158,000. Jacob Schiff and Mayor William R. Grace opened the Fair and the crowds swarmed around the candy store, the flower stands, the restaurant, displays from schools, a wickerwork stall staffed by Trustee Lyman Bloomingdale and thirty-four women, and all the other delights. There were some remarkable sights. The Japanese Garden had "pine and fir trees, a bamboo house, a miniature grove of palms and ferns, a Japanese home, a life-size wax figure of Montefiore in an armchair, together with booths for the sale of vases, plaques, screens, fans, and decorative articles, embroideries, portieres. . . . The effect . . . heightened by electric lights, which gleam with all the fairy splendour of a scene from the Arabian nights."

On the last Saturday evening of the Fair, 7,000 people were crushed together among all the delights, and the doors were closed to newcomers for half an hour. All the newspaper accounts emphasized the beauty of the young women who did most of the selling. One reporter estimated that of the 999 who took part, 999 were belles.

Charity, however, was more than raffles and chaperoned flirtations. Mrs. Simon Borg, the first President of the Ladies' Auxiliary Society of the Home, thought deeply about purposes. In a speech to the National Council of Jewish Women, her topic was "A Practical View of Philanthropy." She spoke about the needs of the discharged hospital patient: "It surely has occurred to every one of you that if voluntary aid were forthcoming, and many of these convalescents who are no longer under the jurisdiction of the hospital, were looked after for a week, or perhaps two, before they make any attempt to go to work, they might in numberless cases, be saved from becoming chronic invalids." The Auxiliary, under Mrs. Borg's thoughtful direction, experimented with social services, with occupational therapy and education for patients. Mrs. Simon Baruch was more traditional in her approach, forming the Montefiore Home Flower Mission to bring flowers and music to the bedside.

As hospitals became more acceptable to the middle and upper classes, paying patients became more important to many institutions, but not at Montefiore. Few families were able to survive the financial impact of chronic illness; few could pay the bills for months or years of care. Paying patients were a tiny minority as long as Montefiore provided only care for the chronically ill. Most of the money for the Home came from individual contributions, but as expenses mounted, the Directors began to look for other sources.

In 1879, the Hospital Saturday and Sunday Association, later to be known as the United Hospital Fund, was organized "to obtain benevolent gifts for the hospitals of New York . . . also to further economy in management and to coordinate and extend the work of the hospitals." The Home joined the Association in 1887, receiving a subsidy of $976.63, which covered 5 percent of the year's expenses. A few years later, the Association insisted that Montefiore must include the word "hospital" in its title if the subsidy, which was by then the largest received by any member agency, was to continue, and the institution became "The Montefiore Home, a Hospital for Chronic Invalids," the first of many name changes to come. The negotiations with the Association began a long history of involvement with outside funding agencies, private and public. Montefiore was never to receive more than a small percentage of its income from people able to pay their own bills. In the meantime, the city of New York recognized the role that Montefiore played in the care of the indigent sick and gave $1,000 to the Home, following with $500 each year until the turn of the century.

The Trustees recognized that the patient under treatment was not the only person affected by chronic illness. Jacob Schiff took the fees that he received as executor of the estate of his friend Julius Hallgarten, and set up the Hallgarten Fund to support the families whose breadwinners were in the Home. Those two notions, seeing the patient as a member of a family system and the need for the economic and emotional support of that family, were also to remain central to the way Montefiore was to function.

The Trustees also set up, each of them contributing $50, the Discharged Patients and Climatic Cure Fund. Mr. Schiff described the Fund's purpose: "Without this resource, we should be compelled to turn those who leave our care penniless upon a cold world at a moment when they are little prepared to stand its hardships or to forthwith gain a living. The assistance we are thus enabled to give these discharged patients enables them to tide over the time from their discharge until they can find some means of support, or in some cases to seek a milder climate, where a better chance of recovery is afforded them." The discharged patients were inclined to travel. In 1890, seven of them used money from the fund to travel to Europe, one went to Chicago, one to Cincinnati, one to New Haven, one to Jerusalem, and five to Vineland, New Jersey.

Several organizations provided services for the patients and the Home. The Young Ladies' and Gentlemen's Society arranged entertainments, usually with amateur talent. Singers, instrumentalists, and children who had learned to recite the sentimental verse dear to the Victorian heart were brought to the Home to provide distraction. The Young Ladies' Sewing Society worked hard supplying the Home with linens and "garments for the inmates," but in the spring of 1888 merged with the newly formed Montefiore Home Auxiliary Society, which, under Mrs. Simon Borg, continued sewing while experimenting with services designed to meet the broadest non-medical needs of patients. The Auxiliary began a formal education program for the younger patients (in 1890, there were five patients under ten years of age and twenty-eight aged from eleven to twenty) and those activities for patients of all ages which later were to be provided by a professional Department of Occupational Therapy. Patients were first involved in the task of repairing the Home's supply of clothes. (Because most were able to walk around or at least move in wheelchairs, they dressed in normal day clothes, not in nightgowns.) In 1902, the Auxiliary set up an "industrial workshop for the production of ornamental iron work and other articles," which became, according to Mr. Schiff, "a source of much interest to the unfortunates, whose lives drag wearily along and to many of whom this opportunity for healthful and easy labor is most welcome." A few years later, the Auxiliary set up one of the first professional Social Service Departments in a hospital in the United States. (The first was at Massachusetts General.) This role of initiating services that later became part of the routine hospital structure remained the most important function of the Auxiliary at Montefiore.

CHAPTER

3

The New Home:
A Place for Research

The Board of Trustees always looked upon the Avenue A address as temporary. The small house could not possibly hold all those who needed care. In 1885 there were 121 applicants, of whom only 49 could be admitted; in 1886, 116 applied and 43 were admitted; in 1887 only 25 of the applicants could be taken. Many of those who could not be accommodated in the Home were treated in their own homes and given a living allowance for themselves and their families.

A large, imposing building was planned in an area filling up with Jewish institutions. The Home for Aged and Infirm Hebrews stood at 105th Street and Ninth Avenue, the Hebrew Orphan Asylum was at the top of a hill at 138th Street and Tenth Avenue, and the Hebrew Sheltering Guardian Society was at Eleventh Avenue and 151st Street.

Simon Baruch urged the Trustees to include the most up-to-date equipment in the new building. He spoke to them of the great possibilities for scientific research: " . . . the opening of our new buildings will form an era, not only in the history of our institution, but also an era in the history of the treatment of serious forms of chronic disease in this country."

The new Home was to reflect not only the growing research ambitions of physicians. The technology of heating and lighting and plumbing that was changing America's homes and hotels was also changing the hospitals. Chamber pots were necessary under sickbeds as long as outdoor privies were the rule. The Montefiore that lay ahead had not only steam heat to keep patients warm in winter but indoor flush toilets and hot and cold running water in all the bathrooms. Dr. Baruch had all the facilities for hydrotherapy. Nurses could keep patients and bed linens clean. There were laundry rooms in the basement and dormitories for the "laundry ladies" in the attic.

The new Home, with 140 beds, was a complex of separate buildings, called pavilions, in line with the latest theory of hospital construction, designed to limit the spread of infection as well as to separate the sexes. A main building of four stories was used chiefly for administrative purposes. The cellar, kept cool by its depth underground, contained a wine room, a vegetable room, a room for keeping ice, and general storage space. Above this level was the basement, with the dispensary, the smoking room, the kitchen, the laundry and drying rooms, the employees' dining room, the refrigerator, and two flush toilets. The ground-level floor connected with the two other pavilions and held the reception room, the synagogue, the doctor's room, a sitting room for the patients, their dining room, planned to hold about half of them—the number who were not totally bedridden and could gather together for meals—and a room for the Board of Trustees, which had a toilet and washbasins attached.

On the second floor (also connected with the other pavilions) were the doctors' and matrons' bedrooms, each with attached parlor, bathroom, toilets, and washbasins. The assistant doctor's room and those of the chief male nurse and chief female nurse had only washbasins. Here also were the linen, clothing, sewing, and recreation rooms. On the third floor was a dormitory for thirty-five employees with attached toilets, bathrooms, and washbasins. (The bathrooms and toilets throughout had tiled floors and enameled tile wainscoting.) On the same floor was the operating room, fifteen feet square, with a bay window for light and a concrete floor. Procedures may not have been as up-to-date as the architecture. A photograph taken the year the new building opened shows the operating room in use with three doctors and the patient on the table, apparently undergoing surgery, all in business suits, the patient even wearing boots. There was an elevator in this building, and dumbwaiters connected the kitchen with butlers' pantries throughout the complex. A sun room about fifty feet long was built with glass sides and glass roof.

All the buildings had pipes for gas and were wired for electric light, bells, and telephones as well as being equipped with speaking tubes. Steam heat, supplied by burning coal, kept a temperature of 66° to 68° F. during the winter. The Home was built with as little use of wood as possible and with fire escapes suitable for the use of invalids. The fire-fighting capacities of the city were in a primitive state, and employees were formed into a fire company that drilled once a week and in case of emergency fought conflagrations under the direction of the engineer with fire extinguishers and a hose.

In addition to the administrative building, there was a pavilion for male patients and one for women. Each had one room for eight beds. The other rooms held one, two, or three beds—an arrangement that provided for considerable privacy.

The new Montefiore Home opened in 1889 as the first hospital in the United States in which hydrotherapy was a regular and systematic part of treatment. This, Baruch felt, accounted for the dropping of the mortality rate to half what it had been in the old building. In the first year uptown, seventy-one cases were treated with water. Of these, eight were listed as cured, thirteen as improved and discharged, twenty as improved but remaining in the hospital, ten as unimproved, and ten as dead.

In his book *An Epitome of Hydrotherapy for Physicians, Architects and Nurses*, the doctor described some other treatments at Montefiore. Patients suffering from arthritis were suspended in hammock baths for periods of from five to sixteen hours, the temperature being kept between 88° F. and 100° F. The results were favorable: "Patients who for years had to take aspirin [after the Bayer Company marketed it in 1898] or some other form of salicylic acid to quiet their pains and give them rest could get along quite comfortably with no medication at all."

For paralysis agitans "our routine medication was hyoscine scopolomine, which in some instances had to be given thrice daily in order to obtain relief. When the bath treatment was begun all forms of medication were stopped, and patients who for years would crave their hyoscine could do without it very well."

But water, to Simon Baruch, was not just a treatment for those patients who today might be seen as fit candidates for psychotherapy or physiotherapy. For him, water was the answer to almost all ills. He recommended it for, among other problems, cases of typhoid fever, sunstroke, pneumonia, pulmonary tuberculosis, neurasthenia, influenza, and gout. His suggested methods of application included not only whirlpool baths for injured limbs, but intestinal irrigation (after an enema) for infantile diarrhea, catarrhal jaundice, Asiatic cholera, renal insufficiency, and dysentery. One of the charms of water seemed to be that it could be applied in so many ways—wet compresses, wet sheets wrapped around the patient, tub baths, shower baths, or jets of water squirted at the sufferer.

The Trustees and Dr. Baruch still did not see eye to eye on admissions policies and the goals of the institution. Although he had persuaded them to build the extensive hydrotherapy facilities and other improvements in the new building, he complained that "despite the fact that in the planning of the building I had insisted upon a costly and perfectly equipped rest room, heated in winter and opening to the south, it proved impossible to induce these desperate people to submit to discipline by reason of the mistaken kindliness of the directors, whose chief aim was claimed to be to smooth their dying days."

His annual reports gave him the opportunity to lecture the wayward Trustees. In 1896, he wrote: "The methodical application of physical remedies, such as rest, exercise, diet, baths, and fresh air and the exclusion of drugs, except for urgent palliative purposes, has resulted in great good to the patients. But not alone has this beneficent result been brought about, but there is in addition recorded a saving of fifty percent in the bills for the past fiscal year, despite the increase of actual medical work." Opposition had come not only from the Trustees. As President of the Medical Board, Baruch had found it necessary to engage in "constant agitation of the subject with the members of successive house staffs."

The Columbia University College of Physicians and Surgeons appointed Baruch professor of hydrotherapy, although the college later discontinued both the chair and the subject. The more obvious properties of water were not lost on Baruch, who was responsible for the building of free public bathhouses in Chicago and New York. The "Apostle of Bathing," as he became known, was the first president of the American Association for the Promotion of Hygiene and Public Health, which he helped to organize in 1894. In his later years, his son Bernard provided him with an income so that he could devote his full energies to the propagation of the gospel of hydrotherapy. When he retired from Montefiore in 1910, Dr. Baruch felt that the Trustees had come along far enough for him to present them with his portrait, inscribed: "As a Token of Cordial Regard and High Appreciation of Their Earnest and Courteous Cooperation During His Service."

There were, of course, other doctors serving the patients at Montefiore. A larger house staff was necessary, consisting of a senior and a junior house physician, both supervised by the attending physician and surgeon. The senior house physician visited all the wards every morning and every afternoon, examining each patient at least once a day. Once weekly he made an inspection of the whole building and reported the results to the Executive Committee of the Board of Trustees. He was expected to "examine all applicants for admission, and write a minute account of their history, symptoms and general condition" and to discuss the patient with the junior physician before submitting the application to the Executive Committee for their decision. To discharge a patient, he had to have the consent of the Executive Committee, or in case of an emergency, the Superintendent. The patients were safe from his wrath since he could "not discipline nor permit any patient to be disciplined except with the permission of the Chairman of the Executive Committee." He could complain to the Executive Committee in writing about any patient.

The junior physician was a very busy young man. He lived at the Home and was never allowed to be away from the Home for more than half an hour at a time—although on special occasions he could be given permission by the senior physician for "a longer absence, not exceeding half a day." He would not have had time for more extended absences. His other duties included accompanying the senior physician on all his rounds, and every night visiting each patient, making sure that all the attendants on the wards were on duty and giving them final instructions for the night. He kept all the medical records, made up all prescriptions, and supervised "their distribution and administration." He was expected to "enter into a book all prescriptions . . . and all extra food and stimulants ordered for patients." He had charge of all the instruments and medical supplies and was "responsible for their condition." He kept a list of the instruments and made sure that none of them left the institution except for repairs, and also kept a list of all the visits made by the medical staff. For several years the pattern followed was that of the junior physician succeeding the senior physician, so that each had two years of experience at the Home.

Each ward had at least two nurses during the day. They began work at 7 a.m. and finished at 8 p.m., to be succeeded by the night nurses, who wore "slippers or other noiseless shoes." The female nurses were dressed in white caps and aprons and the male nurses—again on the scene—in white jackets.

For many years, the Trustees of Montefiore referred to Mount Sinai as "our mother institution," and indeed, that was very much the relationship. Many of the patients came from the older hospital. Many men served on the boards of both institutions. Jacob Schiff himself was a member of the Mount Sinai board from 1879 to 1885. Isaac Wallach, who organized the

Grand Fair of 1886, was president of Mount Sinai from 1896 to 1907.

Many physicians were on the consulting and attending staff of both hospitals, the great men from Europe as well as the American-trained. Many Montefiore doctors were graduates of internships and residencies at Mount Sinai, including Josephine Walter, who in 1885 became the first American woman to complete a regular hospital internship and who later became a consultant in gynecology at Montefiore.

Under Dr. Baruch's leadership, the Home was attracting some of the best doctors in the city to donate their time for patient care, teaching, and research. Carl Koller, who had been a friend of Freud, discovered the value of cocaine as a local anesthetic in eye operations in Vienna in the same year that Montefiore opened. By the end of the decade, he was living in New York and serving the Home as an attending ophthalmologist. On staff as a neurologist was Bernard Sachs, who in 1887 published his identification of amaurotic family idiocy (Tay-Sachs disease), a hereditary disorder transmitted as a recessive trait responsible for a metabolic defect and chiefly affecting children of Eastern European Jewish background.

Charles Loomis Dana, another neurologist attracted by the opportunities for teaching and research at Montefiore, was a professor of diseases of the mind and nervous system at Postgraduate Hospital and later a professor of diseases of the nervous system at Cornell University Medical College. His *Textbook of Nervous Diseases and Psychiatry for the Use of Students and Practitioners of Medicine* went through ten editions between 1892 and 1925.

The attending staff had increased threefold since the opening of the Home. Eighteen physicians now made regular triweekly visits to the patients. As well as general physicians there were surgeons, ophthalmologists, neurologists, and laryngologists. As Dr. Baruch said: "The appointment of a more numerous staff of specialists was necessitated by the long distance to the institution, and the exacting character of our cases. This subdivision of the work conduces to its more perfect execution and utilization for scientific purposes." The Home had other advantages for research projects. The patients were poor, desperate enough to accept any form of treatment, and confined to the institution for lengthy periods of time, allowing for long-term observation. Jacob Schiff was interested in scientific progress and prepared to spend his money and use his contacts in Europe to obtain the most up-to-date information and discoveries.

Tuberculosis was the most prevalent disease at Montefiore. Of 304 patients treated in 1890, at least 126 were consumptive. The staff was always alert for any news of progress in treatment, especially from Berlin, from where, eight years before, had come Robert Koch's announcement of the identification of the bacillus. In 1890 the great day came. Koch told the Tenth International Congress of Medicine in Berlin that he had produced both a cure and a vaccine. The substance—temporarily called "Koch lymph," since the great man refused to reveal the ingredients—could, according to its discoverer, both protect against the disease and save those already infected. The news was hailed all over the world by patients and doctors alike. Sufferers flocked to Berlin; all the sleeping cars on the trains were booked for months ahead. Koch's tremendous reputation ensured against all doubts.

The magical preparation was tuberculin, made by boiling, filtering, and concentrating a culture of tubercle bacilli. In the long run, tuberculin was proved not to be a cure. The value of Koch's discovery was in its usefulness as a diagnostic tool. Injected into a person who is not infected with tuberculosis, tuberculin has no effect. Used on an infected person, tuberculin will produce a local inflammation at the site of the injection and, in some cases, fever. Tuberculin, in modified form, is still used to test for tuberculosis, a positive reaction indicating that the subject had been infected at some time, although the disease may not be active.

An indication of how closely the staff and Trustees at Montefiore kept in touch with medical advances in Germany is that on November 16, 1890, the Executive Committee of the Board of Directors resolved that: ". . . the medical staff be requested to advise the board of directors prior to Sunday next what steps can be taken to secure prompt trial at this Institution of Dr. Koch's newly discovered method for the cure of consumption and that medical staff be further advised that if it be found requisite to send of their number to Berlin in behalf of the Institution the expense will be provided."

Mr. Schiff discussed the whole matter with sixty-year-old Dr. Abraham Jacobi, who was not to become a member of the consulting staff at Montefiore until five years later, but had long been an influential figure in American medicine. Jacobi left his native Germany after imprisonment during the revolution of 1848 and became a pioneer in the new specialty of pediatrics, founding the Children's Departments at Mount Sinai and German Hospitals and teaching "the diseases of children" at Columbia. He encouraged the Montefiore interest in tuberculin, and Schiff sent a Dr. Einhorn "to go to Berlin and make investigations." The quest was successful. Perhaps Dr. Einhorn had hopes of becoming chief investigator, but that was not to be. At a meeting of the Executive Committee held on December 25, 1890, "Mr. Schiff read a letter which he had written to Dr. Einhorn requesting that gentleman to hand the Koch lymph which he had brought from Europe to Dr. Baruch."

Simon Baruch was grateful for the chance to participate in "this greatest therapeutic investigation of all time" but retained a skeptical attitude to the value of tuberculin as a cure.

As always, Dr. Baruch was aware of the danger to patients and did his best to protect them: "Realizing the enormous import of this experiment and desiring not to subject any of our patients to needless risks, I gave personal attention to it. Fully equipped and prepared by observing the results in Mount Sinai Hospital, I began a series of cautious injections." He was also aware of Koch's reputation: "Coming from so authoritative a source and bearing upon such vital propositions, the utmost care was exercised in order to exclude all bias or other prejudicial element."

The twenty-eight cases for the experiment, selected by Max Rosenthal, the hardworking resident physician, included males and females in the first, second, and third stages of tuberculosis. Some had improved, some remained the same, and some grown worse under the routine treatment at Montefiore, which consisted of "good food, fresh air in abundance, exercise, rain-baths, cod liver oil, creosote, and anodynes if needed." Creosote is today used to preserve wood. Twelve of the female patients were turned over to a doctor who, after three weeks, became dissatisfied with tuberculin treatment and abandoned the experiment.

Dr. Baruch took personal charge of the daily treatment of the other sixteen for six weeks. By the end of that time, he knew the individual reaction of each of them to tuberculin and "other conditions ensuring their safety." He allowed Dr. Rosenthal to continue their treatment under his supervision. The experimental program of tuberculin injections began in December 1890 and continued through the summer of the following year, serving, according to Baruch, "to bring out in more pronounced lines the great value of Hydrotherapy in the treatment of phthisis."

He was not the man to run a truly scientific test. So completely committed to hydrotherapy as a treatment that he was unlikely to discover worth in any other, he also lacked the attitudes and skills that would have permitted or enabled him to set up an objective experiment of a comparison between one group of patients receiving tuberculin injections and one or more groups receiving other forms of treatment or none at all. Such a format does not appear to have occurred to the investigator. All the patients about whom he reported received a variety of treatments: hydrotherapy, cod liver oil, creosote, and tuberculin injections.

Once Koch had identified the tubercle bacillus, a diagnosis of tuberculosis could be confirmed by testing the patient's sputum for the presence of bacilli. In the new Home, the test was routinely done with entering patients suspected of infection with tuberculosis. There was also some understanding of the infectious nature of the disease. The Trustees had invested in the grand new building partly to allow for some separation of the tubercular patients from the others. J.S., one of the experimental subjects, was a thirty-year-old male nurse in the Home who showed obvious signs of tuberculosis. He had several hemorrhages and the bacilli in his sputum were "abundant." He was given cod liver oil and creosote for several months but did not improve. When he began tuberculin treatments he had a severe reaction, fevers going up to 102 degrees. His cough improved under the treatment and he gained five and a half pounds. Under testing, the bacilli were "not so abundant." There had been an improvement, but the bacilli indicated that he was still an active tuberculosis case. Nevertheless, J.S. was allowed to return to nursing patients at Montefiore.

Another of the patients was a female nurse, and the records suggest that contracting tuberculosis may have been recognized as one of the hazards of working in the Home: "She was constantly engaged in the wards, in which her mother was also a nurse. She began to lose flesh while at work; cough and expectoration were pronounced and she had two slight hemorrhages." After twenty-one injections and daily rain baths she was able to resume work as a private nurse, "feeling perfectly well." In her case, however, no bacilli were found in her sputum at the end of the treatment.

Looking back, it is difficult to assess exactly what either doctors or Trustees comprehended about the infectious nature of tuberculosis. They knew Koch's work well, and they had sought out his tuberculin. There are many steps between the acquisition of a piece of knowledge—here the identification of the bacillus of tuberculosis—and the working out and implementation of all the procedures that are ultimately based on that piece of knowledge.

The diagnostic value of tuberculin was tested. One patient was regarded as nearly recovered because his cough and expectoration practically ceased and his temperature remained normal. For diagnostic purposes, he was given one milligram of tuberculin on December 16, 1890. His temperature went to 102 degrees and when his sputum was tested the telltale bacilli were found. The injections were continued and cautiously increased until April 29, when he was given thirty milligrams, with scarcely any reaction, and no bacilli were found in his sputum.

A diagnostic coup was made in one of the two cases in which the tuberculosis was located elsewhere than in the lungs. The patient whose spine was affected did not improve. The other was the oldest patient in the group, a fifty-year-old Russian who two years before suffered from inflammation of the middle ear and the mastoid and was operated on several times in hospitals in New York City. When he came to Montefiore, he had a hard swelling on the left side of the neck, extending from his spine to his throat, very disfiguring and forcing him to hold his head at an angle "15° out of the perpendicular." He had five "fistulous canals"—holes—running down into his neck, one opening into his mouth. Ulcers spread over the entire left side of the neck and swollen glands formed a hard compact mass. His speech was unintelligible because of all the swellings, and he was very weak, bedridden, and "constantly moaning." The discharge from the ulcers was "exceedingly offensive," and all kinds of antiseptics were tried in an effort to deal with the stench.

Dr. Baruch strongly suspected that the infection was the result of tuberculosis. Other doctors disputed this. In spite of the danger of provoking a fatal fever, Baruch decided that a correct diagnosis was important enough to risk the use of tuberculin. Five milligrams were injected and the patient's temperature shot up to 102.4 degrees. The diagnosis of tuberculosis was confirmed. The surprise, even to Baruch, was that the patient began to improve. The ulcers healed entirely. He was able to move his head and speak clearly. Almost all the fistulas cleared up. The man stopped complaining, became cheerful and hopeful of entire recovery, and was able to leave the Home for short periods of time. This was the one case where Baruch, although he had used tuberculin originally purely for diagnostic purposes, felt that there may have been some curative power at work.

In his annual report of 1893 Jacob Schiff spoke of the continuingly increasing demand the growing numbers of immigrants placed upon the Home. The staff at the Home also noticed that many of the patients in the new building were recently arrived immigrants from Eastern Europe, "Russians as to nationality and tailors as to occupation," as Leo Ettinger, one senior house physician, remarked. Of two hundred and twenty-two treated in the course of one year, seventy-three were from Russia, eight from Rumania, nine from Poland, thirty-three from Hungary, fifty-one from Germany, and twenty-five from Austria. Twenty-six actually listed their occupation as tailor and there were enough shirtmakers, pressers, and cloak makers to confirm Dr. Ettinger's perceptions.

Other judgments were made about the patients' mental or moral condition. The young house staff, many of them trained in Europe, had come under the influence of some of the various schools of medicine, which placed great reliance on overt physical signs of interior states of mind. In this classical age of observation and classification of symptoms, physicians had great hope that every physical or mental state possessed a distinct sign, easily identified by the acute diagnostician.

The Montefiore staff read the medical books that sought physical indications of mental ills or aberrant behavior. They looked hard at the incoming patients for the stigmata of degeneracy. The records are full of such notations: "degenerate ears," "large asymmetrical head," "face asymmetric," few of these having any possible connection with the disease for which the patient was admitted.

Some of the routine questions had not been asked in earlier days. All adult males, regardless of the problem that had brought them to the Home, were questioned about masturbation, "venereal excess," and "venereal infection." Women were not asked these questions.

The symptoms of venereal disease produced moral judgment. A patient who arrived with tabes dorsalis, the late stage of syphilis, in which the spinal column and sensory nerve trunks deteriorate, was described as "not moderate in pleasures and habits—a strong smoker and a fast liver."

The nineteenth-century neurologist could not see inside a brain or a nervous system. He could only look at the way in which a patient walked or sat or used his hands. The absence or presence of particular reflexes was critical. Many a doctor achieved textbook immortality by identifying and naming a reflex of diagnostic importance.

The necessity of relying on outward appearance produced, in turn, an overreliance on the method. Eager house staff at Montefiore tested every possible reflex in patients. A computer bank could be filled with the details of the knee jerks and chin jerks and absences thereof between 1890 and 1900.

The staff had other concerns about incoming patients. They worried that, in an age of crowded tenements with one toilet to a floor—or a yard—and few bathrooms, their charges were not very clean. The transmission of disease by infection was accepted as a theory. The pathways of infection were not always clear, but head and body lice were common enough to require constant vigilance. Newly admitted patients were given baths and clean garments. Their own were destroyed unless a friend or relative agreed to take the old clothes away at once.

The records indicate a consideration of the patients as people, with careful attention to the patients' own words, often written down meticulously. E.A. came to Montefiore on November 18, 1897, at the age of seventy-six, after ten years of life in the United States. According to the record, he complained of "Leibschmerzen and Kreuzschmerzen"—body pain and back pain. The account goes on to say that "diese Schmerzen Kommen & gehen"—the pains come and go—and when E.A. ate or drank he suffered "heftige Schmerzen"—heavy pain—and "oftmals Diarrhea."

Both patient and doctor were more comfortable with German than with English. The record goes on to say that "patient sick since few months" and "had never bloody discharges." E.A.'s chin jerk was absent, but his triceps jerks, knee jerks, and Achilles' jerks were all active.

The staff was also careful to watch for bedsores. Immobility creates pressure, and pressure cuts off the blood supply to cells, which die, and bedsores are the result. They are uncomfortable, painful, ugly, and can be deadly if neglected and allowed to become infected. The only prevention is constant vigilance and care. Some patients must be moved as often as every two hours.

Well-placed pillows can help. "Air cushions" and "ring cushions" were frequent gifts to the Home. Once bedsores develop they must be cleaned and protected to allow healing.

Not everybody was confined to bed, and many responded to care. Those who could, were encouraged to be up and dressed. Many were able to move around in wheelchairs. The average length of stay in 1893 was 353 days, which meant that, since many died within days or weeks of admission, many lived for years. They made lives for themselves inside and outside the institution. L.B. entered Montefiore in 1891 and stayed for thirty-eight years. The death certificate showed that L.B. suffered from generalized arteriosclerosis, hypertension, cardiac hypertrophy and dilatation, and combined posterior and lateral column disease of the spine of unknown origin.

In 1901, a hormone extracted from the adrenal glands was first isolated. Adrenalin is the trademark by which it is now known in the United States. Epinephrine is the generic name. At Montefiore, Drs. Jesse Bullowa and David M. Kaplan used hypodermic injections of adrenalin chloride to treat asthma attacks. The paper they published in *Medical News* of October 1903 shows patient care and research at Montefiore definitely entering the twentieth century. The knowledge so painfully accumulated in the United States and Europe during the preceding hundred years was finally bearing fruit in specific treatments for specific conditions.

In their paper, the doctors first list all the varieties of care formerly given at the Home to a patient suffering an asthmatic attack, an enumeration that includes more methods that suggest roots in medieval tradition than any with scientific sources: "Fumes were inhaled from the various powders the bases of which are stramonium, belladonna or hyoscyamus with potassium nitrate. Opium and morphine were given by mouth, rectum and hypodermatically. In some cases relief was afforded in one-half to one hour, but only when doses large enough to produce stupor were administered. Frequently when the narcotic effect wore off the attack would return. Chloral and the bromides were given, but their action was not prompt and not always satisfactory. Nitroglycerin and hyoscine were administered. Camphor and ether were given hypodermatically. A combination consisting of antipyrin and caffeine was used. Chloroform anesthesia was resorted to in some obstinate cases in order to produce general relaxation; often the attacks would return with the wearing off of the anesthetic. Inhalations of oxygen were tried. Emetics were exhibited, cupping and mustard footbaths were resorted to. Silver nitrate injections into the vagus region were used. Adrenalin chloride was sprayed into the pharynx without satisfactory results. In fact, almost all the text book methods were exhausted without much benefit to the patient."

The doctors discussed the necessity of stopping attacks so that the patients' lungs would not be further weakened: ". . . during the asthmatic attack . . . there is an obstruction to the escape of air from the air vesicles and the air vesicles are overdistended. As a result of the obstruction the walls of the air vesicles are forced to expand their elasticity upon an air-cushion, so that, finally, they are overstretched, thus losing part of their elasticity. . . . The many distended vesicles with their non-elastic walls enlarge the lungs to such an extent that they cause an increased intrathoracic pressure, producing an enlargement of the thorax and the characteristic barrel-shaped chest."

They wrote about two then current theories "accounting for the obstruction in an asthmatic attack." The most popular was that "the bronchial obstruction is brought about by a spasm of the circular muscles of the bronchi." Since, however, antispasmodic drugs had not been useful during attacks, they inclined to the second theory, that "the obstruction is caused by a turgidity of the bronchial mucosa." Both theories happened to be correct: during an asthmatic attack the muscles around the small bronchi (the air passages of the lungs) contract and there is a buildup of mucus.

Their first case was a seventeen-year-old girl, born in Russia and admitted to Montefiore in 1900: "In 1898 patient caught cold while bathing. Two weeks later she had a typical asthmatic seizure lasting two days and three nights. One month later she had another attack lasting three days. Another spell, which was observed at New York Hospital, lasted three days. Since then attacks of asthma recurred at intervals of from one day to two months. These attacks are usually preceded by malaise, pallor of the face and a few wheezing rales upon deep inspiration. Then the dyspnea [labored breathing] becomes more and more marked, the mucous membranes become congested, the face and extremities cyanotic [blue] and cold, the wheezing and noisy breathing is heard at some distance from the bed and the patient's distress is evident. These attacks return at irregular intervals and are apparently influenced by various conditions, such as atmospheric changes, dust, smoke, physical or mental exertion, menstruation, constipation, and, at times, without any evident cause . . ." An attack was once brought on by a visit to relatives in bad weather.

The patient lost twenty pounds in two months as the result of the attacks. After successful treatment with hypodermic injections of adrenalin chloride she regained the pounds as quickly as she had lost them. The sophistication of the tests available to the medical staff is indicated by the analysis made of her blood during attacks: "hemoglobin, 80 percent; red blood corpuscles, 4,800,000; white blood corpuscles, 8,600; differential count of blood white corpuscles gave polynuclear neutrophiles, 38 percent; transitionals, 8 percent; small lymphocytes, 6 percent; large lymphocytes, 8 percent; mononuclear leucocytes, 10 percent; eosinophiles, 26 percent; basophiles 4 percent."

The patients who benefited from the new therapy covered a range of ages and occupations: a sixteen-year-old seamstress, a thirty-seven-year-old housewife, a sixty-year-old peddler, and a sixty-three-year-old tailor, "an excessive smoker and moderately alcoholic." Some of these patients and others suffered side effects, but "these sensations never lasted longer than ten minutes and have never been noticed to any marked degree when the drug has been administered in the proper dose."

Dosages and precautions were specified: "With fresh preparations of the drug 3 to 6 minims of the 1 in 1,000 solution, hypodermatically, cut short the asthmatic attack, usually with-

out disagreeable sequelae. It is worthwhile mentioning the fact
that solutions of adrenalin chloride deteriorate from exposure to
light and air, and that the dose must be increased accordingly."
(The next year, adrenalin was to be synthesized and thus solutions and dosage became more standardized.)

The paper refers to English, American, German, and Russian
studies of asthma and ends with thanks for "his generosity, encouragement and advice during the progress of their work" to the
house physician, Dr. Siegfried Wachsmann, the man who was to
become one of the most important medical directors of Montefiore.

This was undoubtedly one of the first clinical uses of adrenalin anywhere. In the history of Montefiore, this was one of the
first successful specific medical treatments. Adrenalin was not a
cure. Asthma is still a disease that can be treated but rarely
cured. Adrenalin, however, was a treatment for asthma specifi-
cally. It was not a general, all-purpose treatment like hydrotherapy. It was not a treatment designed to relieve pain or build
up the general condition of the patient. Adrenalin treated the
special symptoms of asthma.

Surgical treatment had always been specific. The surgeon
removed an infected limb or a cancerous breast. Most medical
treatment everywhere was still general, but the first steps
toward specific treatments for particular conditions were being
taken.

4

Anarchism, Zionism, and Fusion: The Politics of Tuberculosis

Meanwhile, Montefiore experimented with one of the most successful non-specific treatments of all time. The search for a means of direct attack on the bacillus that causes tuberculosis was to continue for more than fifty years, but along the way, a method was found of building up the body's own defenses to repel invasion.

Throughout the nineteenth century, doctors urged upon their patients who were rich enough to afford the treatment, the benefits of a change of climate for tuberculosis. The British fled their own damp and foggy island for the sunshine of the Riviera. Others favored the bracing mountain air of Switzerland. Tuberculosis was often a slow-moving disease that took years to kill. It was also a disease against which, in the early stages, the natural defenses of a healthy body were often effective. Rest, fresh air, good food, all helped the young and vigorous fight off infection and there were many recoveries or long periods when the bacilli lay dormant. In 1884, the same year in which the Montefiore Home opened, the sanitarium movement came to the United States when Edward Livingston Trudeau opened a cottage on

Saranac Lake for the care of consumptive patients. For almost seventy years, fresh air, rest, regulated exercise, and good food were to be the accepted and frequently successful treatment for early cases of tuberculosis. Professionals and public alike disagreed about the details of the formula, arguing about whether the freshness or the coldness of the air was more important, and the most desirable proportions for the rest and exercise mix. Many different climates and landscapes were recommended: mountains, seashore, desert. Warm, cold, and dry atmospheres had their champions. Those who could not afford to travel slept on their own porches or in their backyards.

The Trustees at Montefiore also subscribed to the change-of-climate theory of treating tuberculosis and almost from the beginning provided funds for a few patients discharged as "improved" to travel to some place thought to be healthier for their lungs than crowded New York City. Some went back to family in Europe, some went to California. In the spring of 1895, one of the Trustees, who had lost a daughter to tuberculosis, Lyman G. Bloomingdale, of the department store family, made a donation toward the setting up of a sanitarium in the country to which the lighter cases of tuberculosis at the Home could be sent. Jacob Schiff matched the donation and the Trustees began to plan.

They did not rush into a decision. Most of the money was invested until a suitable location was found and the interest was used to send patients to various areas to test the effects of country air. They were sent to Woodbine, Alliance, and Norma, all small towns in New Jersey that were already sites of Jewish settlement.

In Russia, Jews had been forbidden to own land, as was the case in other countries that codified anti-Semitism into law. One of the results of anti-landowning decrees was an earlier urbanization of Jews than of the surrounding peasant population and their accidental training in the skills for survival necessary in a Europe and an America where city dwelling was the wave of the future. Another, opposite result was the creation of that longing for land and the practice of agriculture that was to give such strength to the kibbutz movement.

The traditional appeal of the United States to the European emigrant was that of a place where cheap land was available, the symbol of the pioneer being the covered wagon going West carrying a family about to establish its own farm. During the Civil War, Congress passed the Homestead Act, opening up vast areas of the plains to small settlers.

The notion of sturdy Jewish farmers plowing their own acres also appealed to the philanthropists who financed much of the emigration. To the nineteenth-century imagination, cities were seen, often quite realistically, as places of physical and moral danger. Cholera and typhoid epidemics were still frequent, housing for the poor barely touched by sanitation laws. The countryside looked healthy by comparison. In the case of Jewish immigrants, cities held the additional threat that anti-Semitism tended to increase as the size of any Jewish community grew.

The Montefiore Trustees, however, seem to have been influenced by the school of thought that saw a connection between altitude and the cure of tuberculosis, and when they ultimately bought land it was not in the flatlands of New Jersey but at Bedford Station, "the highest point in Westchester County" which was also "entirely free from mosquitoes and malaria" and, forty miles from New York, "within one and a half hours' railroad ride from the city," so that patients could be transferred easily and doctors from the Home could visit frequently "at slight cost to the institution."

In June 1897, a 136-acre farm that came with "a substantial farmhouse . . . together with barns and other outhouses" was purchased. Alterations were made to make the farmhouse suitable for fifteen patients, and a bathroom and "hot-water heating apparatus" were installed. Farming was to continue, as part of the therapy for patients, and as a source of food for both the Sanitarium and the city institution. Indeed, the Trustees hoped that the farm would make the Sanitarium self-supporting. Mr. E. C. Powell, a graduate of Cornell University, was appointed agricultural superintendent and proceeded to buy tools and equipment. Mr. and Mrs. Daugird were appointed superintendent and matron of the Sanitarium.

Fifteen patients, all men, were selected from those in the

Home and sent to the Sanitarium for observation and treatment. There they began a rather strenuous schedule, being expected to "attend to the domestic arrangements of the house, such as the making of the beds, setting of the tables, sweeping of the rooms, clean windows, they also attend to the pump and heating apparatus and any of the incidental work around the house. The tailors repair the clothing, the painter does some odd jobs of painting and the carpenter assists with such carpenter work which is necessary in the house, and, under the direction of Mr. Powell, they assisted in such light farm work as hoeing, weeding, husking corn, picking apples, etc."

Within eight weeks, the Sanitarium was supplying milk and eggs to the Home, and the Trustees hoped that the taste of country life would persuade discharged patients to settle permanently away from the crowded tenements of New York City. In these early days, not all the patients at the Sanitarium were consumptive. Others with asthma or "nervous diseases" were sent there in the hope that they too would benefit from rural life.

A gift of $5,000 from Mr. and Mrs. Lewisohn, in memory of a dead son, paid for half the cost of a new pavilion to house twenty-four patients. The wooden structure was built with wide porches and many windows to provide the fresh air that was so important as a part of the treatment. The dormitory was designed with twelve beds along the lower walls and another twelve on the gallery that ran around the upper part of the two-story-high room, an arrangement that made for the maximum circulation of air and the minimum of privacy. Only male patients were admitted. A deep well was dug and water was carried to the pavilion by a windmill, supplying enough for drinking, the heating system, and the hydrotherapy that continued to be an important part of any Montefiore treatment.

During the first year there was no physician living at the Sanitarium. If a patient began spitting quantities of blood, a messenger was sent three miles over country roads to Mount Kisco to bring back a doctor. The staff organization was changed when, in September, Dr. Henry Herbert was appointed as resident physician and superintendent of the Sanitarium. Dr. Herbert's supervision produced, by the end of the next year, a statistical report which provides a detailed picture of the work at the Sanitarium. By August 31, 1899, sixty-seven men were treated, of whom forty-two were discharged after an average stay of six months and twelve days. About a third of the patients were married. They came from Russia (thirty-one), the United States (thirteen), Austria–Hungary, Germany, and Rumania. About a third of the discharged were apparently cured and almost half were improved. Gains in weight were most important since doctors had few other ways of judging whether their patients were getting better. Group photographs show individual weight gains meticulously noted on the borders. Dr. Herbert reported that, in his first year, of the thirty-eight inmates he studied, twenty-eight gained in weight, four lost, and six remained stationary, the highest weight gain being twenty-six pounds.

Other kinds of scientific research were conducted. On July 1, 1899, a United States Weather Bureau was established, enabling Dr. Herbert to report mean temperatures for July, August, and September. Thus, the Sanitarium was ready with the data for comparative studies of the effect of climate on tuberculosis, and "during the year a laboratory was established to do microscopical work," so that samples of sputum no longer had to be sent down to the city for examination.

The farm was flourishing with five horses, one colt, twelve cows (ten milkers), one bull, two calves, a heifer, two hundred and fifty chickens, and sixty ducks. Fifty acres were under cultivation, and with seventy tons of hay, two hundred barrels of potatoes, two hundred bushels of oats, and twenty-five hundred head of cabbage on hand, the Sanitarium was able to sell some of the surplus potatoes, as well as apples, hay, red beets, beans, four hundred and fifty-five ears of sweet corn, and tomatoes. Milk, butter, and eggs were in good supply and one hundred and thirty-five tons of ice were cut from ponds on the grounds and shipped to the city.

The success of the Sanitarium convinced the Trustees that

they could cope with the problems of overcrowding at the city Home by expanding the country buildings and sending all consumptive patients to Bedford. They began to plan for a facility that would hold one hundred and fifty patients and cost $200,000.

The new facility, with "an imposing frontage of 419 feet," consisted of four separate wings, two on either side of the administration building, to which they were connected by a ten-foot-wide corridor. Women were to occupy two wings, the men the other two. (Children were to form a large proportion of the patients, but no separate accommodations were planned for them.) There was apparently some doubt about too much fresh air. While the buildings stood on a "commanding position on an elevation overlooking a beautiful valley," they were "sheltered in the rear from the distressing and harmful north winds by a rising bluff." In spite of the sheltered position, temperatures inside the airy wards frequently fell to 40 degrees Fahrenheit. An expert landscape gardener, Otto Buseck, was called in to lay out the grounds. All the buildings were lit by electricity from a specially installed generator, and "advanced scientific plans" were adopted for the proper disposal of all sewage. The Lewisohn Pavilion was converted to a synagogue, and Mr. Lewisohn gave $40,000 for the maintenance of one of the female wards in memory of his wife. There were some delays in construction. At a meeting of the Medical Board on October 17, 1899, "the Building Committee reported that erection of the new home had been postponed because cases of malaria have occurred at the country branch. It was requested that the Building Committee investigate this matter and try to discover whether there is any stagnant pool near the proposed site for the new building."

Throughout the long life of the sanitarium movement, arguments raged in medical circles about the amount of rest that was most helpful to the patient. At times even reading was forbidden. In Bedford, however, at the turn of the century, work was part of the prescription, valued as much because it was good for the character as for the lungs. Dr. Alfred Meyer, "Con-

TO REORDER YOUR UPS DIRECT THERMAL LABELS:

1. Access our supply ordering web site at **UPS.COM**®
   or contact UPS at 800-877-8652.

2. Please refer to label #0277400801 when ordering.

0277400801   RRDR

sulting Physician of the Country Sanitarium," wrote admiringly that "the prize pumpkins, cabbages, radishes and ears of corn would have done credit to a country fair" and "the value of such a regime to the patients themselves is simply inestimable."

Dr. Herbert was also pleased, reporting that three quarters of the cases showed improvement, the results "proportionate to similar figures from other sanitaria, even including those for the well-to-do classes." At a per capita cost of 76.8 cents per day, three hundred and seventy-seven patients were treated in the first year in the new buildings. Many of the patients had additional complications to their physical conditions, including alcoholism, arthritis, arteriosclerosis, asthma, appendicitis, cirrhosis of the liver, diabetes, and on through the alphabet to vitium cordis (a heart abnormality) and varicocele (a varicose condition of some of the veins of the testicle). Surgical procedures were now done at the Sanitarium. Dr. Herbert himself performed a thoracotomy (a surgical incision in the wall of the chest) and an operation for caries (decay) of the bone. Adenoids and tonsils were removed, ribs and knee joints resectioned, and procedures undertaken for empyema (accumulation of pus) of the gall bladder and two cases of fistula in ano (an opening on the body's surface near the anus which may or may not have penetrated through to the rectum).

Patients were followed up after they left the Sanitarium. Sixteen were known to have died after discharge, and of forty-five others who responded to the inquiry blanks sent out, fifteen said they had improved, seventeen were in the same state of health as when they left, and thirteen reported that they were worse.

The next year, Dr. Herbert was replaced by Dr. L. Rosenberg, and his reports, while as carefully statistical as those of his predecessor, give a fuller account of life at the Sanitarium. A new dining room was built for the employees and the old one turned over to the nurses and orderlies for recreation. The farm continued to produce. The hilly approach to the Sanitarium was "completely rebuilt and regraded, . . . the sides of the road terraced and sodded, and a substantial stone wall erected alongside the abutting field." The poplar trees, planted two years before, made "the ascent to the Sanitarium heights a shaded avenue of gentle grades."

Dr. Rosenberg's tables reveal, as Dr. Herbert's did not, that many of the patients were children. Two of them were only six years old in his first year, and twenty-one (out of a total of 365) were under the age of sixteen. His wife, to whom he referred as "Mrs. Dr. L. Rosenberg," organized a school and a reading class for the children. The school was popular. Boredom was always a great problem for Sanitarium patients and administrators alike. Young adults joined, and soon the classes were also held after the regular weekly services in the synagogue. The children started their own newspaper and a drama group, which gave an open-air performance for the benefit of the Bedford Fire Department. Entertainments were also provided by volunteers from the city, and the staff gave lectures in popular science on Friday evenings.

Despite the new buildings, the Sanitarium could not accommodate all the people who applied for admission. The Ladies' Auxiliary supplied three tents, each with two beds, that were used to take care of six extra patients in the summer. Old horse-drawn streetcars were also brought to the Sanitarium and used as dormitories for some men. Dr. Rosenberg's house staff consisted of four medical officers, three "graded and salaried" and one unsalaried but in line for promotion in case of a vacancy. The total staff, medical and non-medical, including ten nurses and orderlies, added up to about forty-eight.

Rectal temperatures were taken twice a day, and a reading of over 100 degrees Fahrenheit resulted in a bed-rest order. The urine of all incoming patients was tested for signs of diabetes.

The patients were served three "generous" meals a day, and bread and milk were available between meals and at bedtime. In accordance with Dr. Baruch's teachings, shower baths were a regular part of the treatment for male patients and those who did not take showers were required to take a "cleansing tub bath" once a week. In the interest of cleanliness, beards and moustaches were trimmed and sometimes shaved off entirely.

The disposal of the highly infectious sputum was a problem

at all sanitaria. At Bedford, those who spat on floor or ground were "instantly" discharged. In the early years, each patient was given a glass bottle with a metal screw cap into which to spit. The bottles were emptied into a large metal pail where the orderlies mixed it with sawdust. Twice a day the whole mess was dumped into a special furnace and burned and the pails washed with hot water. The sawdust, bought from a local mill, cost twelve dollars a year.

Fresh air, abundant food or even "hyperalimentation" or over-feeding, and hydrotherapy were the basic treatment, but in 1905 Dr. Meyer reported to the annual meeting of the National Association for the Study and Prevention of Tuberculosis on some of the drug therapies at Bedford, aware as he was that sanitaria were "peculiarly the object of faithful attention by pharmaceutical houses" anxious to try out new products. He was not impressed with a combination of eucalyptus, sulphur, and carbon recommended for inhalation and was cautious about experiments, feeling that "it would appear preferable in most cases to select for trial such patients as have derived all the benefit attainable from the usual hygienic, dietetic, atmo-spheric, and hydropathic measures and whose condition has become stationary under the sanitarium physician's eye." At Bedford, continuous fever was treated with soluble silver, various unspecified coal-tar preparations, and spongings. Two patients who were found also to have malaria were successfully treated with quinine.

Dr. Meyer was also concerned about the uncertainty of diagnosis, knowing, as he said, that many sanitaria were filled with misdiagnosed cases of emphysema, asthma, and bronchitis. (The problem of a certain and speedy diagnostic tool for tuberculosis was not to be easily solved. In 1980, the labs at Montefiore were still struggling with the riddle.) During the first six years of work at Bedford, Meyer experimented with tuberculin injections in forty-five patients, but he was not sure enough of his results to publish them. He suggested his own method of percussion of the patient's chest. Instead of tapping two or three times, he hit the chest twenty to thirty times to produce a "series of sounds . . . wave-like in character in its rise and fall," reminding the doctor of "nothing so much as the waves due to musical notes produced by the piano tuner when tuning the instrument." A comparison of sounds on each side of the chest allowed a guess at the state of the lungs. With professional diagnosis so uncertain, persuading the public of the danger was difficult, especially if there was no cough, "which for the layman" was "the sine qua non of pulmonary tuberculosis." In the circumstances he looked upon the early spitting of blood as "a fortunate accident, a blessing in disguise" if the reluctant patient was thereby persuaded to accept treatment.

Dr. Rosenberg was plagued with a problem that was to haunt future sanitarium administrators—"the reasonably rigid separation of the sexes." The wards were divided, male and female, but most patients were out of bed, dressed and active most of the time. One hundred and fifty of those 365 patients were between the ages of sixteen and thirty and reminded constantly of how short life could be. The help of Mr. Isaac Blumenthal, a Trustee, was sought in dealing with one aspect of the problem. There were not enough shade trees near the women's dormitories. Mr. Blumenthal financed the construction of a "handsome and commodious pavilion" where female patients could seek shelter on sunny days and thus avoid the temptation of seeking shelter on that part of the grounds reserved for males.

There were other aspects of patient behavior with which Dr. Rosenberg was unsympathetic. One hundred and ninety of his charges were Russian-born. They spoke Yiddish, a language that he found strange. Indeed, he had trouble believing that it was a true language, and referred to it (as did many of his contemporaries in the United States and Europe) as "jargon." There were two literary societies at the Sanitarium. Dr. Rosenberg reported that one conducted meetings in English, the other in "jargon." He also noted that Mr. Schiff, apparently more tolerant, or more aware of reality, had made a gift of "191 volumes of jargon books."

Yiddish was often the language of the political discussions that helped to pass the long hours. Many of the patients had been politically active in a Russia approaching revolution; many of them were part of the labor movement in the garment factories of New York City, one of the first solidly unionized industries. "Tailor" was the most common occupation listed by men, "operator" the second. On the roster of female occupations appear "operator," "tailoress," "millinery," "seamstress," "dressmaker," "cloak maker," "shirtmaker," and "shirtwaists." The connection between poor living conditions and tuberculosis was heavily publicized by the public health movement. Politically minded consumptives were likely to blame the capitalist system for both their disease and their housing and not likely to feel grateful to the rich for the charity that provided medical care. The fact that the clothing factories in which the Russian Jews worked were often owned by the same German Jews who founded the hospitals and sanitaria did not lessen the conflict. Administrators at the Sanitarium easily confused political discussion and patient complaint, seeing in both the specter of anarchism, currently haunting official minds on both sides of the Atlantic. Dr. Rosenberg wrote to the same Board committee asking for the discharge of ten men who seemed a danger to the discipline of the Sanitarium: "It will be readily understood by all intelligent lay-men how fatal to success in the treatment of tuberculosis is a state of dissatisfaction and rebellion against the salutary discipline of a sanitarium; added to the pardonable bitterness which many patients feel against the hard fate which has made them victims of a dreadful disease, is the despair of betterment which goes with the belief that they are being underfed, maltreated and neglected. *Our patients are easily inflamed by adroit ranters, as they variably attribute their state to anything or anybody but the disease from which they suffer.*"

Dr. Rosenberg also worried about the patients who insisted on leaving against his advice. In 1904, thirty-nine patients were discharged for "infraction of rules," while one hundred and eleven left at their own request. The Sanitarium was isolated, patients felt far away from family and friends, and worried about those they had left behind. Both they and their families were new to a strange land. The claims of family were the most common reasons for leaving before the doctors thought patients were ready. Additionally, patients with tuberculosis often have periods of feeling very healthy even though the infection is still present.

He was also anxious about the places to which they returned, the streets and tenements of the crowded city. Most of the patients came from lower Manhattan, east of the Bowery. There were nine from Clinton Street, seven each from Madison and Monroe, six each from Delancey, Eldridge, and Essex, and so on through the sad litany. He wrote to the Board: "Unfortunately, the majority of our inmates are with difficulty convinced of the advantages of life in rural communities or the healthfulness of light agricultural pursuits, and these usually return to their former insalubrious surroundings and occupations." He was aware of the problem of finding employment in the country and in at least two cases he was able to help. As usual, he wrote of himself in the third person: "Opportunity recently made it possible for the Superintendent to appoint two former inmates to positions in the institution, the one as nurse, the other to a post of responsibility in the executive office."

He urged more sources of suitable employment, writing in 1908: "There should be subsidiary or co-operating enterprises in connection with sanatoria for the treatment of consumption, whereby suitable and hygienic employment would be assured those who have withstood an attack and will have to start out again with a revised mode of living and vocation."

The dream of widespread Jewish settlement on the land did not seem realistic to Dr. Rosenberg: "Farm-colonies, fairly successful in some parts of the world, will not do for our own particular charges. They require for their success first of all the enthusiastic co-operation of the patients, some bent for a rural life and agricultural pursuits. Our inmates are intensely urban in their instincts, with a long heritage of city-dwelling forefathers behind them to accentuate their distaste for country life and occupations; and they have not the physique necessary for success in even the lighter forms of farm operations."

Mr. Schiff was not to be so lightly discouraged from his dream of a population of Jewish farmers. The next year Dr. Rosenberg's annual report began: "In a previous report the Superintendent referred to the perplexing problem of the after-care of patients discharged from the Sanitarium, expressing particular regret that . . . our charges were not such from which a self-supporting agricultural class could be recruited. This somewhat disheartening view of the situation was not shared by some members of the community. . . . Accordingly, with the approval of your Sanitarium Committee and the financial support of your Honorable President [Mr. Schiff] . . . a suitable tract on the farm was set aside and divided into fifty patches having the capacity, under intensive cultivation, of about the average family vegetable garden. A trained instructor, a graduate of the Doylestown Agricultural School, was put in charge of the work, and the members of resident staff cooperated by giving the venture that close medical supervision which every undertaking with tuberculous patients necessitates."

The patients apparently shared Dr. Rosenberg's lack of faith in market gardening, but he endeavored to reassure the Board of the success of the experiment, by which "it was possible to demonstrate to an exceedingly skeptical set of people that this form of work could be shorn of all imaginary drudgery and severity and be made a source of pleasurable exercise and . . . that under intelligent management it affords an absolutely practicable mode of earning a livelihood under circumstances highly advantageous for individuals whose concern must ever be the conservation of restored health."

Other questions concerned Dr. Rosenberg. The number of applicants to the Sanitarium tended to be three fifths male and two fifths female, so the number of beds was divided in the same proportions. Women, however, remained longer at the Sanitarium. The average length of stay was 162 days for women and 136 days for men. Dr. Rosenberg's explanation was that men had greater responsibilities. This was true in the sense that men were more likely to be the financial support of families. In a typical year, 512 patients were treated, of whom 307 were male and 205 female. Of the men, 132 were married, and of the women, only 67. The statistics, and the doctor's observations, also indicate how decisions about treatment were often made more on economic than on medical grounds.

Dr. Rosenberg worried about the patients' teeth. "Most of them have some defects requiring immediate repair, many have very few and some even no useful teeth left." He felt this was particularly important when good food, and therefore the ability to eat, was such a vital part of the treatment. Some dental work was done at the Sanitarium, but Dr. Rosenberg felt that a better method would be to have all the work done in the city while the applicants waited for admission.

Accurate diagnosis was often difficult, as Dr. Rosenberg acknowledged. The early symptoms—cough, loss of weight, slight fever—could be the result of other problems. Sorting out cases of "doubtful diagnosis" became a time-consuming activity at the Sanitarium. In 1912, 126 of these cases were admitted. Of these, "68 were discharged as 'non-tuberculosis,' after a varying period of observation; 43 were subjected to the tuberculin test, and, reacting thereto, kept in the institution for three months as a rule; 25 failed to react, and [were] included in the 68 above enumerated; 11 refused to submit to the tuberculin test, 7 left before complete observation could be made, and 4 children . . . still under observation; 36 were discharged without resort to tuberculin, the evidence being insufficient to justify such a procedure."

Koch's tuberculin, which had been tested by Simon Baruch as a possible cure or preventive vaccine, was now firmly established as a diagnostic tool. Tuberculin was to retain its usefulness in that role but with many changes in attitudes toward the information it conveyed. Today tuberculin is used for mass screening, the first step in testing a whole population, and a red rash on the patch of skin on which tuberculin has been placed means only that the person has been exposed to tuberculosis, not that the disease has taken hold. Only a few of those who react positively to tuberculin prove, after X-rays and sputum culture, to have tuberculosis.

At the Sanitarium in 1912, a positive reaction to tuberculin was taken to mean that the patient had tuberculosis. At least the test did release thirty-six (if they believed the results and the doctors) from fear and from months of treatment. By the next year, the Sanitarium had advanced to more precise standards with its own X-ray department "under the immediate charge of Dr. Leopold Jaches and Mr. Thomas Scholz . . . carefully organized and its equipment perfected . . . so that the service has been of great value in clearing up most matters of diagnosis and a very great help in interpreting and controlling the effects of the new treatment."

Diagnosis was still an uncertain matter and "dubious" was added to the table of annual statistics to cover "those cases in which the evidence, while insufficient to justify a diagnosis of pulmonary tuberculosis, is still of such a nature as to forbid its unqualified rejection."

The "new treatment" to which Dr. Rosenberg referred was surgical. For many years, some cases of tuberculosis were described as "surgical" if infected glands or kidneys or limbs could be surgically removed. In 1913, a procedure was introduced at the Bedford Sanitarium to prevent an infected lung from working in the hope of restricting the spread of infection. Artificial pneumothorax was first suggested by an Italian, Carlo Forlanini, in 1882. The lungs are normally wrapped in a double membrane, the pleura. Between the two layers of membrane is a very thin layer of fluid. If air, or some other gas, is forced between the pleura the difference in pressure forces the lung to collapse. Forlanini first experimented by pumping nitrogen into the pleural cavity in 1882. Dr. Rosenberg felt that the year 1913 "was made epochal" by the use of artificial pneumothorax at Bedford.

The technique helped some patients, although no one was sure of the reason. "Rest" was always a magic word in the treatment of tuberculosis, and Dr. Rosenberg invoked it to explain that the treatment had "the object of effecting a partial or complete compression of the diseased lung, much as inflamed or injured joints are immobilized by various means for the purpose of producing that functional rest essential for a cure."

In spite of his horror of anarchism and socialism, Dr. Rosenberg planned changes in the factories where his discharged patients toiled: ". . . we should endeavor to reduce the extreme of effort now put forth by the average worker under existing conditions of competition, and also make possible a wholesome and simple dietary, and sanitary centers for amusements or self-improvement or social intercourse."

He was trying to provide "in a small way . . . a solution of this vast question. A number of intelligent ex-patients are employed in the Sanitarium in various capacities."

The farm itself continued to flourish, producing, in 1911, milk, eggs, apples, strawberries, cherries, muskmelons, watermelons, rhubarb, parsley, chives, and thirty-six different kinds of vegetables, running at a loss of only $3,110.35 that year.

There were two streams of medical thought in the last half of the nineteenth century that between them were to bring about great improvements in the general health of the public in the new century. There were those who pursued the quest for specific causes of infection and specific means of prevention or treatment of disease. They hoped to duplicate Pasteur's feat of creating a vaccine from the infecting agent.

Others concentrated on cleaning up the environment, providing sewers and good housing and good food to create a healthier population. The two schools of thought were not necessarily opposed. The sewers drained away the germs that caused cholera or typhoid fever. The pasteurizing of milk killed sources of infection. These interrelationships were not always obvious to contemporary combatants. The sanitarians—the public health advocates and environmentalists—feared that attention paid to the germ theory of disease would distract attention from the need to clean up the streets and houses and plumbing. They feared also that taxpayers would be less willing to pay for improvements, businessmen less willing to shoulder their share of the burden of providing decent housing for workers, if they felt that an easier answer could be found through vaccines and germicides.

Tuberculosis was the disease that united the two schools of

thought—although the Pennsylvania Society for the Prevention of Tuberculosis, formed in 1892, was careful to exclude from membership people who did not believe that the disease was contagious. But the successful fight against tuberculosis was to be fought by people who believed that it was caused by a particular bacillus and also believed that living conditions were important in spreading the contagion. The National Association for the Study and Prevention of Tuberculosis was formed in 1904 to engage in "not only the scientific study of the disease of tuberculosis, but a study of all its relations to man, social and economic, and all measures for its prevention, eradication and cure."

The public was barraged with propaganda in all the sophistication of twentieth-century technology. Pamphlets were written and distributed. Movies were produced and shown on the walls of tenements or in parks on hot summer evenings. Thomas Edison lent his talents to the production of melodramatic silent two-reelers such as *The Temple of Moloch*, which showed a wicked factory owner, unwilling to clean up the dust in which his coughing workers were forced to labor, finding enlightenment when his beloved daughter came down with the dread disease. Schoolchildren were enlisted in the campaign to educate their ignorant parents in the principles of good nutrition and sanitary housekeeping. Tuberculosis was the first disease on which was brought to bear the full American talent for publicity and fund raising.

This was the era of progressive reform in American politics; 1906, the year in which a Pure Food and Drug Act was first passed in spite of intensive lobbying from manufacturers more interested in easy profit than in the public health. That same year, Teddy Roosevelt first used the word "muckrakers" to describe the journalists who were using the new national mass-market magazines like *Collier's* and *McClure's* to expose the evils of unbridled private enterprise. New York City had embarked on that long cycle in which political control was to swing not so much between Republicans and Democrats as between the forces of corruption and the forces of reform. A complicating aspect of this pattern was that reformers in New York City were usually interested in clean government, which was usually interpreted to mean less expensive government. The opposition always enjoyed spending money and was ever prepared to spend money on services, whether direct or indirect, to the latest immigrant group which could be cajoled into registering and voting. These same politicians and their friends were also prepared, whatever the era, to spend money on building highways and hospitals and schools and bridges, which provided jobs and services to the needy while also providing great wealth to the not so needy. The poor, enjoying the fruits of corruption, were not always quick to appreciate the benefits of reform government and its economies.

Seth Low was a hero of reform politics in New York City when public health was high on the agenda of progressive politics at the local and national levels. Twice mayor of Brooklyn, president of Columbia University, he was elected mayor of New York City on a fusion ticket—another traditional and perennial device of New York reform politics.

Mayor Low, after cleaning up the police and education departments, improved the air by forcing the New York Central Railroad to change over to electricity from coal within the city limits before he was toppled by the regrouped forces of Tammany. He was an appropriate speaker for the 25th Anniversary celebration of Montefiore, the institution so heavily engaged in the fight against the disease regarded as the greatest issue in public health, the disease most likely to be tamed by efforts to provide good housing, food, air, and the education of all. Jacob Schiff said of Seth Low that he laid "the foundation for good municipal government and good municipal government includes social work of the very character that we [at Montefiore] are doing ourselves."

The Board of Trustees constantly urged the city of New York to take action on various public health matters, to build sanitaria for poor consumptives, to control the manufacture of contaminated snuff, to increase the subsidy paid to Montefiore.

The festivities marking the 25th Anniversary took place in the

"New Ballroom" of the Hotel Astor on October 26, 1909, at eight-thirty in the evening, with a rather grand musical program provided by an orchestra from the Symphony Society of New York. The roster of speakers, ignoring all the other medical conditions with which the medical staff struggled, talked about tuberculosis, the disease that had popular appeal and political significance. Seth Low urged: "Every man in the city of New York, when he casts his ballot, either this year or any other year, for the election of city officials, ought to ask himself, in the form of conscience, by what vote can he do most to help reduce the ravages of tuberculosis."

The beginning of the kind of assistance that Dr. Rosenberg urged for the recovering sanitarium patient came about with the formation in 1910 of the Joint Tuberculosis Committee by representatives from the Free Synagogue and United Hebrew Charities. The committee "undertook to give adequate super-vision and care in the home to a number of families, members of which were suffering from tuberculosis." Forty-nine families, with seventy-nine cases of tuberculosis among them, did quite well under the care of the committee. There were no cases of infection in other members of the families; only 15 percent of the cases suffered any relapse and of these all but one were brought back to an arrested state. The committee reported that "the home conditions were bettered and in the great majority of cases the economic conditions were much improved."

The next step was to compare these results with a control group, families of patients which were not receiving special care. Seventy cases were discharged from Bedford Sanitarium six months to a year before the investigation started. Fifty-two percent were in worse health than when they were discharged and 30 percent of the families had other members who had become infected. The comparison suggested to the committee that "the sanitarium method of turning patients out into the world, partially restored to health and without any further supervision, is not a wholly adequate instrument."

The Joint Committee was expanded to include Montefiore, each body contributing funds. The Home was to give "up to fifty dollars per patient; the Free Synagogue ten thousand dollars per year; and the United Hebrew Charities what it would normally allow its families." An additional $20,000 was collected from the community for the work of the committee.

The approach taken was revolutionary in that "the procedure and theory of care pursued . . . makes the family, not the patient, the unit." The new committee took over fifty-three cases from the old committee and added patients as they were discharged from Bedford. There was a "social investigation" of each family under the care of the committee. The entire family was then examined by Dr. G. Kremer, who was a "specialist in nose, throat and lung diseases." A social service nurse visited the family regularly and undertook "the improvement of hygiene" by instructing the mother "in the proper care of the home and diet for the family." The nurse also took care of any sick member of the family. If housing conditions were unsuitable, the family was moved to "a more sanitary tenement but always such as it should be able to afford." The Board of Health agreed to provide dental care for the school-age children. "The well-known gynecologist Dr. Jellinghaus" volunteered, and three other doctors gave emergency services in the Bronx, Manhattan, and Brooklyn.

Experience showed the committee that patients should not go back to full-time work for an extended period after sanitarium treatment. The Jewish Free Employment Bureau helped the committee to find light work for ex-patients. Farming does not seem to have occurred to the members as a practical or desirable occupation for their clients. The children of the families were "being equipped for the higher grade industrial activities." Nineteen ex-patients or well members of their families were helped to obtain loans from the Self-Help Fund of United Hebrew Charities in order to go into business for themselves. Thirteen of them became peddlers. The other six set up a dental laboratory, a stationery store, a paint store, a building business, a tailoring store, and a workshop to make school bags. The nineteen loans added up to $3,805. By the end of ten months $566.84 had been paid back. Only two cases were "complete failures."

The committee also set about making arrangements to open a model factory where work was to be graded according to the strength and ability of the patients. Operations were to "be regulated as to conditions, hours of work and rest by a nurse under the direction of a physician, the hope being to gradually return the patients to full-time work and efficiency."

Dr. Rosenberg was delighted with the Joint Committee: "All students of the problem . . . have come to the conclusion that the question is so very much a sociological-economical one that the most enlightened efforts on the greatest possible scale, when limited to purely medical means, must needs fall far short of the desired end—the reduction in the number of cases."

The Sanitarium ran more smoothly, with patients willing to stay until their treatments were complete, because, as the doctor reported, "the work of the committee has been particularly fruitful in disentangling complications arising at home, knowl- edge of which is brought to the superintendent by alarmed pa- tients. All such are promptly investigated and the outcome as promptly reported here, thus alleviating much needless anxiety."

He was "now in a position to make full use of sources of information not formerly at hand, concerning the home affairs of the inmates," and able to "calm those perturbed by ill advised missives from home—an all too frequent episode at the Sani- tarium, often leading to precipitate departures." He made the suggestion that a certain number of beds at the Sanitarium be set aside for ex-patients, who could be sent back for a two-week vacation and observation whenever any suspicious symptoms reappeared.

Fred Stein, the Montefiore representative on the committee, worked with a professional social worker, Edward Hochhauser, to set up the factory, which, they were careful to explain, was "not primarily a means of treatment for tuberculosis" but a "scheme of graduated work after sanatoria or even hospital treatment, under fairly ideal conditions." The workers were ex- patients whose sputum no longer contained the bacilli of tuber- culosis. To the loft leased in the Bronx windows were added and a stairway cut through to the roof to provide for an open-air rest area. Since so many of these ex-patients were experienced in the needle trades (and so many of the philanthropists were in the garment industry), the committee decided on men's shirts and middy blouses as the products of the factory. Workers were paid "not less than the union scale of wages," which added up to no more than $9.00 a week for those able to work a full eight-hour day. The non-patient management team, the foreman (from whom the committee first rented and then purchased the loft) and his assistant (who happened to be his brother), were on salary, together with a nurse, a cook, and a watchman. All workers were examined by a physician every two or three weeks and records kept of weight and the condition of heart and lungs. Blood pressure was taken, a urinalysis done, and orders for any treatment or the number of hours to be worked left with the nurse. A special night clinic was held for patients who worked a full day. The workers paid cost for the lunch prepared on the premises and designed to wean them from the "delicatessen food" to which, according to the committee, they were accustomed. A typical lunch, costing ten cents, consisted of fish, rice pudding, bread, butter, and tea. Some patients also received milk (for which they paid), morning and afternoon.

The committee ended two years with 126 families representing 582 men, women, and children under care—181 cases had been closed; 15 had been dropped because they "would not cooperate"; and 39 more had been dropped with the note that "no constructive work possible with either family or patient or both."

Patients were sent to other sanitaria: Otisville, Sea View Hospital, Ray Brook, Medford, and even Denver, which was rapidly acquiring a large Jewish population and excellent medical services as a result of the belief in its clean air and altitude as therapeutic for all kinds of pulmonary conditions. The factory was also used to keep people out of sanitaria: "One young fellow accepted for Otisville was kept at home, and started working one hour a day buttoning shirts. His hours of work were slowly increased, and at the end of six weeks he had improved sufficiently to work 8 hours a day. During the three months he has been working he had earned $104.00, his condition is improved, he is doing as well as he might have done at the sanitarium, is self-supporting, and much happier than if he had been at an institution."

The workers were carefully watched for signs of fatigue and stress. Another man was "found too weak to work on his first examination, and was told to rest for two weeks. At the end of his two weeks' rest he was permitted to do light work at the factory for two hours a day. This was slowly increased to eight hours, but after working six months the doctor advised that he rest for two weeks. Two months later he had to rest for two weeks again. Since then he has been working a full day, his condition has improved very much and he had gained seven pounds. During the year, since he started to work at the factory, he has earned $332.17."

After twelve years at the Sanitarium, Dr. Rosenberg resigned to go into private practice and was succeeded by Dr. Louis Shalet, who had previously been at the Otisville Sanitarium. Dr. Rosenberg used his annual reports to the Board of Directors to express his disagreements with their policies (especially to the back-to-the-land theory), his worries about the patients, and suggestions for changes. Dr. Shalet was of a different temperament. His reports were brisk accounts of improvements: "a new laundry completely equipped with the most improved electrical machinery . . . new lavatories and baths installed in each ward . . . new steel tables, racks, electrical dishwashing machines, new cork-lined refrigerators . . . diffused light fixtures . . . new all-steel insulated lockers. . . . All available rooms . . . used previously as living rooms, storerooms and for similar purposes are now occupied by beds for patients. This has enabled us to install 44 additional beds. [The Sanitarium now held 225 beds.]" Dr. Shalet did have some requests—all for equipment: movies for the patients, a new X-ray machine, and a "properly appointed pathological laboratory." By the next year, they were all in place—with the addition of dental equipment for the use of the dentist who came up twice a week. The movie projector was installed in the rear gallery of the synagogue. Dr. Shalet turned his attention to the farm. The help's quarters were renovated and a bath and "sanitary plumbing installed for the first time." The walls of the milk room were tiled, a modern milk cooler installed, and steps taken to bottle the milk served to the patients.

Dr. Shalet did not need to lecture the members of the Board. They were agreed on the aims of the Sanitarium. The patients who came to the Sanitarium in 1916 gave more varied occupations than before. There was a stenographer (male), a journalist, a dancing teacher, ten porters, a photographer, and a mechanical dentist. But there were still "52 operators, 41 tailors, and 10 dressmakers." No one dreamed of making farmers of them. For rehabilitation they were offered, not garden plots, but a garment factory in the Bronx.

CHAPTER

5

Moving to the Bronx

The members of the Medical Board at Montefiore complained with gloomy frequency that they were not consulted often enough by the Board of Trustees. At Montefiore, lay control of the hospital remained stronger for a greater length of time than in many institutions. Few of the patients could actually be cured, so that the doctors did not seem to possess great power. The patients were much more dependent for their well-being than those in acute-care hospitals on the kind of non-medical services that the members of the Board and the Auxiliary could provide: entertainment and education, social services and subsidies for families.

The Medical Board made frequent requests for measures aimed at increasing the scientific excellence of the Home in patient care, education, and research. In the spring of 1899 a resolution was passed: "That the Medical Board feel the necessity of having a room set aside and properly equipped for the performance of capital operations, and that they deprecate the necessity of transmitting inmates of the Home to other institutions for capital operations." Laboratories were becoming a necessity in a first-class hospital, whether for performing tests on patients or for research. Montefiore already had a pathologist on staff. At this same meeting, a resolution was passed to consider "the advisability of creating the position of physiological chemist." The position was created and filled by Dr. Phoebus Aaron Levene. Born in 1869 in Russia, receiving his M.D. from the Imperial Medical Academy in St. Petersburg, and continuing his postgraduate studies at the Universities of Bern, Munich, Marburg, and Columbia, he was later to go on to a distinguished career at the Rockefeller Institute for Medical Research.

Now Montefiore had both a pathologist and a chemist without, by the standards of the Medical Board, adequate laboratory facilities. Whoever was the current Chairman of the Medical Board followed the tradition of Simon Baruch in urging the Board of Trustees to do their duty in support of scientific medicine. In 1903, Dr. Henry S. Oppenheimer took the Directors severely to task: "Thanks to your Honorable Board's provision for the Laboratory, we see most excellent work done there, and if your Honorable Board could see its way clear and complete in this department what it has so well begun, there is no reason why we should not look forward to seeing the work of the Pathological Department of the Montefiore Hospital quoted in every scientific journal and the Laboratory known the world over for its record of research. We have such a wealth of material in the Hospital for use and study, that it is the neglect of a great opportunity not to give our able pathologist every facility and help to exhaust its possibilities."

Four years later the Board of Trustees was ready. The combined Laboratories for Pathology and Physiological Chemistry were set up with Dr. Levene in charge of the Chemistry Division and Dr. Harlow Brooks as Visiting Pathologist. And as Dr. Wachsmann proudly announced: "In combination with the Laboratory research work, a special observation ward has been established for the sole purpose of studying the metabolism of suitable cases according to the most rigid requirements of medical science."

Dr. Wachsmann, at the same time, drew a distinction that

was to become more and more a part of the functioning pattern at Montefiore, the "division between the infirmary and the dormitory," between those patients who could benefit from active medical intervention and those who required only custodial care.

The Laboratories and the Observation Ward were established by the Trustees as a tribute to Jacob Schiff with contributions of $40,000, including $5,000 from Schiff. The first year's work cost $2,697.10. The staff consisted of D. M. Kaplan, M.D. (who had worked on the adrenalin experiment with asthma and was now resident pathologist), Leo Kritellar, Ph.D., the resident chemist, and David Manson, assistant chemist. They spent their time on problems that were common in the Home. Observations were made of "twenty-five patients affected with different forms of muscular disease," patients with Bright's disease, and "a group of patients affected with the disease known as spontaneous gangrene." Many of the patients at Montefiore suffered from disturbances of their circulation which cut off blood from their extremities and led to gangrenous rotting of their toes or feet. Dr. Levene's staff came close to the truth when they decided that "the results of the observations seem to indicate that the disease is brought about by the physical condition of the blood vessels, and not by constitutional changes brought about by faults of nutrition."

As the level of sophistication in medical knowledge increased, hospital administration called for greater skills. At Montefiore, the positions of superintendent and matron were traditionally filled by a husband-and-wife team, both usually with little education, since the roles were seen as basically large-scale housekeeping. The members of the Executive Committee of the Board of Trustees were constantly at the Home, checking on details and making most administrative decisions. Hospital administration was not yet seen as a profession. At Mount Sinai, Dr. S. S. Goldwater was slowly developing the theory of a discipline in the subject. No schools as yet offered courses or degrees.

Montefiore's patients were both poor and interesting. Many of the diseases from which they suffered were rare, and those who spent years in the Home were available for observation over long periods of time. After death, they retained their interest when the body's secrets could be laid bare on the autopsy table. An enormous amount of the knowledge built up about illness over the centuries, that basic knowledge which was now fueling the medical revolution, was based on the dissection of dead bodies, a practice carried out over those same years in bitter struggles against social and religious taboos, when many Christians believed in the literal resurrection of the body and Orthodox Jewish belief forbade tampering with the dead.

Years later, Jacob Goodfriend, a long-time Montefiore administrator, remembered Montefiore's record of having the highest autopsy rate in the city, a record maintained by constant effort on the part of doctors and administrators. "Very often, after the doctors had talked to the family, they would send them to me. I may have gotten the permission because I was a layman. I would say, 'What do they want?' And the family would say, 'They want an autopsy.' And I would say, 'Look . . . I don't think I'd give them permission to do that. If they want just a small incision, fine, but make sure I'm there so they don't do anything they shouldn't do.' Then they'd take me along and say to the doctors, 'You can't do a complete autopsy. It isn't necessary. Confine yourself to a small incision.' Look, that's psychology."

To improve the skills of the nurses, male and female, Dr. Wachsmann, the senior house physician, set up classes. Two hours each week were "devoted to instructing the nurses in the elementary branches of physiology, anatomy, surgical dressing, asepsis, sterilization, disinfecting and nursing in acute and chronic diseases, and materia medica, as far as necessary."

Other activities of the hospital were becoming more skilled and more professional, including some duties of the Trustees. From the beginning they had carried out the functions that could be classed as social work: the investigation of the circumstances of applicants, including visits to their homes; the provision of relief to families; finding suitable institutions for those not admitted to the Home; assistance to discharged patients and the search for jobs and housing for them. In 1909, a salaried social worker, a Miss Hallahan, was hired, to be assisted by a committee of the Auxiliary.

In 1909, a Special Committee of the Board again reorganized the medical staff. Dr. Siegfried Wachsmann was already medical director, but he was given "supreme management" of the medical service at the Home. Formerly this authority had lain with the President of the Medical Board. The increasing complexity of medicine necessitated full-time professional direction. Dr. Wachsmann was assisted by a house staff of four physicians and a laboratory staff of three, while the Medical Board of thirty-two "eminent consulting and attending physicians" volunteered their time and advice in a "co-operative capacity." At the Country Sanitarium, Dr. Rosenberg was in charge, with three house staff in training to help him. The beds in both institutions added up to almost 500. (In contrast, Montefiore in 1979 had, in all affiliated institutions, 1,825 beds, with a house staff of 575, a change in ratio from about one resident to seventy patients to one resident to every three.) Each institution also had its own dentist, an innovation for a hospital at the time and an indication of the careful attention that was given to all aspects of the patients' health.

The time was coming for Montefiore to move. The area that was once "the green outskirts of the city" was becoming closely settled. People who lived near the Home were worried about infection and disturbed by other emanations from the buildings. Jacob Schiff explained to the Board: "Criticism is beginning to make itself felt among the neighborhood in which the institution is now located, because we cannot prevent those of our inmates who are not confined to their room from strolling into the adjacent streets nor can we seal up the windows and prevent the moaning and outbursts of physical pain among our sufferers to escape, sometimes to the great annoyance of our neighbors." A move was proposed to the new outskirts of the rapidly spreading city.

On March 13, 1909, Jacob Schiff gave a dinner for the Directors. A motion was passed that the President appoint a committee on sites to find a suitable location "within the northern boundary of the City of New York." By October the committee had found land in the Bronx between Gun Hill Road and 210th Street (bounded on the north by Bainbridge Avenue) and early in the new year bought 162 city lots (about thirteen acres) for $240,000. The city authorities agreed to the closing of parts of one cross street that cut through the proposed site. This enabled the architects to plan for all the buildings to be contained in one superblock.

The old Montefiore Home and the land upon which it stood was sold for $525,000. The Board expected that the cost of the new buildings plus the land would be at least $2 million.

The committee set about organizing a festive occasion. A tent large enough to accommodate 1,200 people was ordered. The Hebrew Orphan Asylum Band was asked to provide music.

Since October 26, the anniversary of the founding of the Home, that year fell on a Saturday, the Jewish sabbath, the ceremony was held on the following Sunday. A regular Board meeting took place, at which Schiff in his annual report made a strong plea for financial support since, in addition to the cost of the new buildings, the Board was faced with an annual expenditure of $300,000 for the support of the almost 1,000 patients who would now be taken care of on Gun Hill Road and in the Country Sanitarium.

At the ceremony Schiff presented to Samuel Kridel, chairman of the cornerstone committee, a silver trowel inscribed with the words of Alexander Pope: "In Faith and Hope the World may disagree, But all Mankind's Concern is Charity."

While the Orphans played the Triumphal March from *Aida*, Kridel laid the cornerstone, which contained "a copper box the gift of Mr. I. Moritz, containing American coins . . . in circulation, daily and Jewish papers, and the last Annual Report of the Home." Simon Baruch was present and that activist physician must have been somewhat disturbed by the poor prognoses for the patients given by some of the speakers. Kridel declared: "Our aim and endeavor is to lessen the burden that many unfortunates have to bear—incurable disease. We establish a home for them and try to make what remains to them of life as pleasant and as free from suffering as lies within human power."

The concerns of the President of the Medical Board, Dr. Felix Cohn, were more directly medical. He saw the purposes of Montefiore as "the humane and skillful treatment of the inmates, the proper utilization of the clinical material, and of the experience gained at the bedside, without detriment to the patient, for scientific development and research, and finally, the educational obligation toward the community."

The buildings were ready to open on November 30, 1913. The New York *Times* called the new Montefiore "the largest Jewish hospital in the world," and the *Herald* referred to the "prominent Jews who inspected the institution." Five thousand people attended the dedication of the hospital set in "the still open country at Gun Hill Road and 210th Street." The *Times* was optimistic that the Home was safe here in the North Bronx, since "the buildings are provided with ample grounds, a 60-foot-wide parkway surrounding the outer fringes of the eight-acre site, with two additional parks, each 125 feet square, in the midst of pavilions, and with white cement walks cutting the green lawns circling the flower beds." The buildings were designed so that further stories could be added later, if growth were necessary.

Dr. Siegfried Wachsmann had revisited Germany to make sure that the buildings conformed to the latest thought in hospital architecture, as well as consulting with that well-known expert on hospital administration, the superintendent of Mount Sinai Hospital, S. S. Goldwater. There were nine buildings in what the *Times* called "colonial style," indicating to the American reading public that red bricks and white columns were involved. A cupola overlooked "the Hudson and Harlem Valleys." A green-painted iron fence ran all the way around to safeguard the neighborhood from the patients. All the buildings were connected by one-story-high corridors to protect patients and staff in transit. The Home was planned for religious observance with a 300-seat synagogue where services were to be conducted in the Orthodox manner without an organ and with "impressive interior furnishings of mahogany amid walls of white and yellow." Two kitchens were provided—one for meat and one for dairy cooking according to the dietary laws—and sets of *milchig* and *fleischig* dishes.

The architecture also recognized the infectious nature of tuberculosis, housing these patients in a separate pavilion with its own laundry and kitchen and a southern exposure with two levels of balconies, the top one set back to allow the sunshine to reach the patients on the lower. Each floor had sixty-two beds, with patients who could walk about on the lower floor and bed patients on the second, all provided with steamer chairs for use on the balconies.

The sickest non-tubercular patients were housed in the five-story, 225-bed central pavilion. Each floor had three large wards and several smaller ones. The doors leading to the balconies were built without raised thresholds so that wheelchairs could be easily pushed through to the fresh air. In the special room for patients suffering from locomotor ataxia (the stage of syphilis of the spinal cord that results in loss of sense of position of the legs and a characteristic gait), a design of footprints was inlaid on the floor to help in teaching patients to walk.

Great care was taken to have everything as easily cleaned as possible. "The plumbing fixtures were selected with great care. . . . In most cases the existing standard designs were changed by the manufacturers to comply with the specified requirements for absolutely sanitary, smooth, round surfaces." The laundry was arranged so that all the material handled flowed in one direction and clean linen would not be contaminated by dirty. All the washers and the wringers were motor-driven and all the ironing done electrically. Indeed, housekeeping and medical technology were both now so advanced that there was danger of one interfering with the other. The electric elevator in the private pavilion was run from a storage battery "to prevent the effect on the fluctuations of the voltage due to starting an electric motor, which would have been detrimental to X-ray work."

Jacob Goodfriend, a stenographer at the time, took the minutes at the meetings of the Executive Committee and the Board and learned how to run a hospital by observation. During the period of planning for the move to the Bronx, he sat and listened and kept detailed records as the members decided how many square feet were needed, how many beds should be ordered, how many pots and pans for the kitchen, the kinds of equipment needed for physiotherapy.

Many years later he recollected: "When they wanted somebody to receive all the merchandise that was delivered before the building was occupied they came to me and at that time I was general clerk and they said to me, 'You're familiar with all the merchandise that was ordered and you helped to assemble statistics. Why don't you take the job as receiving clerk and receive all this merchandise and we'll give you staff after the place is finished and cleaned up and you'll be in charge of placing all this stuff because you know everything about it. You saw from the beginning.' So I got there and after everything was in I was made purchasing agent and after a while they said, 'Why don't you become the steward and make up the menus and so on.' So I became the steward."

Goodfriend also helped with moving the patients, "mostly by cars because most of these patients even if they were bedridden or chairridden they could still be lifted into a car. So mostly it was the automobiles of the Directors and cars that they could get from other people. Undertakers donated their cars and where they had to be transported horizontally, ambulances, but there weren't many of those patients who couldn't sit up."

In celebration of the move, the name of the institution was changed to "Montefiore Home and Hospital for Chronic Diseases." The move to the Bronx changed forever the balance of power at Montefiore. From now on the distance from Manhattan was to be the deciding factor in many issues. As long as Jacob Schiff lived, he was to be an overwhelming presence, but neither he nor any other member of the Board of Trustees, all of them residents of Manhattan, could visit as easily or as frequently as before. The Executive Committee could not make daily visits to talk with patients or check up on the details of housekeeping. The Trustees still waited on the designated corners for Schiff's automobile to pick them up and take them to Montefiore for Board meetings, but their other visits became rare.

Many matters had, of necessity, to be decided by those on the spot in the Bronx. Most not only worked but lived at Montefiore. Siegfried Wachsmann moved into the house that had been built for him on 210th Street, opposite the pavilion housing the tuberculous patients. Jacob Goodfriend moved into the Green House, an old Victorian clapboard that, divided into apartments, was to house generations of administrators. Nurses and the house staff lived in dormitories, as did most of the housekeeping staff.

The day-to-day tasks of administration were huge in scale: the patient care; the buying, storing, preparing, and serving of food; the laundry; the cleaning of the buildings; the supervision of a large professional and non-professional staff. Dr. Wachsmann and his assistants gradually took over more and more of the routine running of the institution with less and less direct attention from the Trustees.

Dr. Wachsmann also accumulated power because he was a physician. The members of the Medical Board lived and worked in Manhattan. A trip to Montefiore took a large part of a busy day. More and more responsibility for patient care devolved upon Dr. Wachsmann and the interns and residents. There was an increase in house staff. When the buildings opened on Gun Hill Road, there were five assigned to those patients. The next year, there were eight, and the next, ten. (The number at the Country Sanitarium remained stable at three.)

Dr. Wachsmann even went so far as to invite women to join the house staff. At a Medical Board meeting in the spring of 1914, Dr. Wachsmann told the other physicians that "such an arrangement would be advantageous in looking after the health of the nurses and female help." In the house staff pictures of 1916, the first woman, Dr. Frances Cohen, is to be seen peering timidly through round spectacles.

The house staff was divided into two sections: one for the

tuberculosis wards and the "general section" for all the other patients. The most experienced residents were known as the house physician and the house surgeon. Below them were seniors, juniors, and externs. The house and senior grades received salaries, and the juniors, a bonus "upon completion of satisfactory services." Hours of duty were 8 a.m. to 7 p.m. At least one senior and one junior were always on night duty. Apart from two weeks' vacation, the house staff were expected to remain at the hospital at all times except for twelve-hour leaves "granted by the Medical Director to the several members of the staff in rotation." Overnight leave of absence was granted only in emergencies.

The medical staff was no longer totally German Jewish. Some Eastern European immigrants were doctors at Montefiore. Maurice Fishberg, "Physician to the Tuberculosis Wards," and also an anthropologist and adviser to Jacob Schiff, was born in Kamenets Podolski, in Russia.

Dr. Michael Ringer was born in a little town on the eastern side of the Prussian border. In 1915, Dr. Ringer had his own private practice in Manhattan, specializing in clinical research on diseases of metabolism, particularly diabetes. "Montefiore," he recalled, "was at the time slowly evolving into an institution of broader scope, from a Home to a Hospital for Chronic Diseases. Dr. B. S. Oppenheimer convinced me of the opportunities it offered for my own program of clinical practice and research. He was the most important influence in the conversion of Montefiore from a Home to a real hospital, and pressed me hard to come to Montefiore in spite of the distance I had to travel daily to get there from my Manhattan office. He promised me a good slice of the budget for research equipment and he delivered. Later, he arranged to get me the privilege of transferring diabetic patients to the private pavilion, where diet and medication could be better controlled. I was put in charge of the clinical laboratory and I selected an enthusiastic group of assistants from the clinical staff, notably Drs. Biloon and Harris and a full-time laboratory assistant. We brought the laboratory up to date. As a group, we were concerned with the metabolic

[9 7]

problems in the department of medicine. When Dr. David Marine became the head of pathology, we retained our independence in research and collaborated with his department in general laboratory service. The scientific tone of the central and west buildings was strongly communicated to the other services. Moses Keschner was a member of the adjunct staff in neurology and gave the patients real dedicated service. He called me in consultation once and I gave the patient a thorough examination, including a complete blood chemistry, which was new for that day. Two days later I brought my figures to him. 'Oh, Ringer,' he said, 'don't give me figures. They don't mean anything to me. Give me your conclusions. That I understand.' Which gives us something of the art and science of medicine around 1915."

Students had always visited the Montefiore wards. Now more formal academic connections were made. Schiff announced in 1916 that "the growing importance of Montefiore Home and Hospital, as concerns medical science, has been evidenced in the past fiscal year through the proposition made by the College of Physicians and Surgeons—part of Columbia University—also by the University of New York and Bellevue Hospital Medical College, for an affiliation of both of those two great medical colleges with this institution, which offer the Directors have accepted, whereupon our Medical Director, as well as certain members of our Attending Medical Staff, have been appointed into the faculty of one or other of the aforementioned colleges."

Three years before, an agreement had been entered into with the College of Physicians and Surgeons for the study of cancer. Several donations had been given by Trustees and their friends for the research, including sums from Mrs. Lewis S. Wolff and Gustave Sidenberg, who "pledged an annual contribution of One Thousand Dollars in memory of his late wife for the purpose of promoting the care of patients suffering from cancer, and to stimulate search after a remedy for this terrible disease."

To fulfill the agreement with Columbia, Dr. Isaac Levin of the Crocker Fund for Cancer Research, who was also clinical professor of cancer research at New York University and Bellevue Hospital Medical College, together with Dr. A. D.

Dakin as consulting chemist and Dr. Nelson W. Janney as resident chemist, were appointed as a research team.

In the first year of the special program twenty cases were admitted, in the second, forty-six. These latter included eleven cases of carcinoma of the stomach, six each of the intestines and rectum, five of the uterus, four each of the breast and peritoneum, three of the lungs, two cases of skin cancer, and one each of the bladder, thyroid, tongue, and esophagus. One "sarcoma" was listed separately. (There are two main types of cancer: "carcinoma" is used for the cancer that arises in the epithelial tissue [the outer layer] of skin, glands, and membranes; "sarcoma" is used for the cancer that grows in the connective tissues, such as bones and muscle. Sarcomas are less common than carcinomas.) Most of the patients were regarded as hopeless and close to death. X-ray treatment was given to sixteen of these; four showed some improvement. Research was done on various diagnostic blood tests in conjunction with the Rockefeller Institute.

Dr. Levin was a strong advocate of radiation therapy, believing: "It is imperative . . . to subject every malignant tumor to treatment by the rays, before the performance of the radical or partial operation. The same holds true of post-operative treatment. The rays may sterilize and inhibit the proliferation of the remaining cancer cells, even if they do not destroy them outright."

Levin strongly, but erroneously, believed that "one of the important effects of radium and roentgenotherapy consists in the formation of an extensive connective-tissue stroma, surrounding and compressing the tumor cells. In skeletal metastases this stroma . . . is transformed into bone." He thought that this connective tissue protected the body from further growth of the tumor. The two ideas resulted in the hopeful, but totally wrong announcement at an annual meeting of the Board of Trustees that "it has been found that in certain bone diseases, radium not alone arrests the disease, but greatly stimulates the growth of new bone. This discovery may be of considerable importance in the rehabilitation of wounded soldiers."

For breast cancer Levin recommended surgical removal of

the tumor by radical mastectomy combined with radium and roentgen therapy, to be given over the operative field, the chest wall, and the whole skeleton or "at least the spine and the heads of both femurs."

He also advocated "in every advanced case, or better still, in every case of carcinoma of the breast, a roentgenographic X-ray examination of the skeleton before the operation. If it is too expensive or difficult to explore the whole skeleton, then those parts should be examined in which metastases most frequently occur, namely the spine and femurs."

Dr. Levin commented on the "frequency with which the primary carcinoma of the lungs is met," apparently unaware that he was seeing the effect of the increased use of cigarettes. He also reported that "Dr. Michael Levine investigated the influence of Roentgen Rays on the carcinoma [crown gall] of plants. The subject is of great practical as well as theoretical importance, since it is proven that plant carcinoma is caused by specific bacteria."

Michael Levine was not a physician but a botanist. For more than thirty years he worked at Montefiore, growing cancerous geraniums and rubber plants and mangel-wurzels, publishing papers fully illustrated with careful photographs of his grotesqueries, funded by many a reputable agency, including the American Cancer Society. His search for the answer to the cancer riddle was fruitless, but his deliberately deformed plants added an interesting flavor to Montefiore's formal gardens.

CHAPTER

6

"Poverty Is a Many-Sided Thing"

The patients, aware of themselves as more than a collection of symptoms, began in 1915 to write about their lives in *The Montefiore Echo*. Contributions were submitted in English, Yiddish, and German; the publication was printed in English, often with a heavy sprinkling of the other languages, under the editorship of Isidor Toplin and Max Messenger, both patients. Letters to the editor dealt with questions both philosophical and practical:

Dear Sirs: Fourteen years ago, at the time of Passover, I chanced to pass the Kireshefsky Hospital in Kiev. At that time I was in danger of losing my life, not from my present ailment, but because I risked my life to save two persons from almost certain death under the hoofs of a team of runaway horses. Now, fourteen years later, a question presents itself: It is again a question of life and death, only the circumstances are altered. What puzzles me is, what feeling prompted me to put my life in danger at that time, when I was young and strong, with the best outlook for a successful future, while now, with no hopes for the future, sick and weak, I desire to live in spite of my ailment?

Some patients made suggestions—or demands:

Dear Sirs: Can I write to you and ask you to give me a little information? I have been a patient of the Home for a number of years. I know that the persons in authority do all they can to make the time pass as interestingly and as entertainingly as possible, but it seems to me that, with all the entertainments that have been given, one thing has been overlooked: that is, moving pictures. We used to have them in the old Home, and can you tell me why it is that in this new Home, which is more complete, "movies" are not shown?

The motion-picture question was frequently raised by both the readers and the editors in the succeeding months, and in June 1916 the campaign was triumphant. The *Echo* printed a letter of thanks to the Trustees.

There were frequent entertainments at the Hospital, featuring both amateur and professional talent, but there were occasional problems in bringing the performers to Montefiore:

To furnish a whole afternoon's entertainment, rendering some fifteen vocal selections, one after another, not only without tiring her audience, but, on the contrary, leaving a distinct appetite for more, is no small feat for one individual to accomplish. Yet such was the task imposed upon Miss Karena Post, soprano soloist, who, on Tuesday afternoon, April 17th, was scheduled to give us a song recital, assisted by Mr. Alberto Garcia Guerrero, which was intended to constitute but one-half of a program designed to include a Marionette show. But fate decreed that the conveyance bearing the Marionettes should break down and that Mr. Guerrero likewise should be unable to attend. Thus it fell upon the shoulders of Miss Post to bear the burden alone, and when we say that she afforded an afternoon's entertainment second to none the patients have ever had, it will be realized that she acquitted herself well.

There was bitter laughter at the plight of the greenhorn, in deliberately humorous pieces:

To my much beloved wife, Becky, you should live and be well with all the children one hundred and twenty years.

First, you shall know, my dear Becky, that I am, thank God, in the Montefiore Home, the fifth day already, and you should also know that yesterday I was examined by two doctors and they tell me that I have tuberculosis. Now, my dear Becky, you need not be worried any more: thank God that I have not got consumption, as I was told at the Board of Health. Of course, you want to know what kind of a disease this is. So I must tell you that this is not such a bad disease, and when I asked the older patients about it, they even laughed and said that with this disease a person can live until his death.

Now, my dear Becky, let me tell you that I have it here very good. You know that at home I used to eat a little piece of meat on Saturday only, and here they give me a big piece of meat every day, that would be enough for you with all the seven children together. And I let you know that we sleep here two men in such a nice, big room that you and I and the seven children could sleep in it, and there would still be room for a boarder.

Now listen, Becky, do you know what I would like? Since tuberculosis is not a disease, and the old patients tell me that a person can live with it until his death, and because it is so nice up here, I should like you and all the children to get tuberculosis. Do you ask why? Because then we could all live here together at the Montefiore Home. I have no more news to write. I kiss you and all the seven children.

The editors took a firm line about the responsibilities of their fellow patients:

A little incident occurred some weeks ago on one of the wards which deserves comment here. A patient had made use of some apparatus and when he had finished with it he made no effort to return it to its proper place. This was called to his attention by another, and his reply was: "Oh, I don't care; let the orderly do it." The one who made this remark was physically able to replace the articles in question, but he seemed to labor under the impression that his sole duty here was just to be a patient and not to make the least attempt to help himself. It is not our purpose to moralize or lecture to our readers, but there is a simple lesson that all of us may learn from this little incident, and we feel it our duty to call attention to it.

Financial support for this large institution was a constant source of concern, even though the expenses, by later standards, were minimal. Jacob Schiff believed that a hospital which cared for so many indigent patients who would otherwise have been public charges was entitled to a subsidy from the city and application was made. The Home was granted 40 cents a day for patients suffering from chronic disease and 90 cents a day for those with tuberculosis. (By 1918, wartime inflation increased these amounts to 60 cents and $1.10.) In 1916, the subsidy amounted to $146,139.42.

The Home continued to receive a subsidy from the Hospital Saturday and Sunday Association, but Schiff had a complaint about the method of distribution, a complaint which would later be echoed by other hospital administrators, referring to other reimbursement agencies: "The Managers of the Hospital Saturday and Sunday Association have adopted a new method of distribution, under which our income from this source has been materially reduced. Heretofore the number of free hospital days was, as we think it should be, made the basis of award from these collections, and because Montefiore does more free work than any other Hospital in this Borough, it has for many years been at the head of the list of beneficiaries from the Hospital Saturday and Sunday collection. Under the changed method, per capita cost is made the basis for the awards, and as we have been able to keep down cost very considerably, we have, because of this, suffered under the new method referred to, receiving only $8,611.98 from last year's collection, as against $10,500 in the preceding year."

The Brooklyn Federation of Jewish Charities donated $7,425.14 on behalf of patients accepted from that borough. The Federation of Jewish Philanthropies, covering the entire city (except Brooklyn, which did not join until 1942), was finally created in 1917 and from then on provided not only an annual subsidy for Montefiore but a third body which Schiff could regularly scold for insufficient support.

At Montefiore, in 1916, the Ladies' Auxiliary raised $10,132.60 and "Friends of the Patients," $20,054.78. Considerable funds ($128,441.65) came from individual contributions from "Benefactors, Donors, Patrons, Members and Juniors." The Hospital held $828,892.28 in endowment funds, most donated by Board members to memorialize a relative, such as Betty Loeb, Schiff's mother-in-law, honored by a $25,000 fund. However, $12,000 came from the Ladies' Bikur Cholim Society and Industrial School Endowment Fund, an organization which had gone out of existence, perhaps from the burden of its duties. (Bikur Cholim—"Friendly Visitors"—denoted a group fulfilling the religious obligation to visit the sick.) Most of the endowment money, $619,500, was invested in mortgages on property in Manhattan or the Bronx. Of the remainder, $50,000 was used to buy 500 shares of the preferred stock of the American Smelting and Refining Company, and the rest was tucked away in railroad bonds, ranging from the Montana Central to the Brooklyn Rapid Transit Company.

Some of the ways in which the money was spent had not changed since 1884. Thus, $599.59 was spent on wines, liquors, and alcohol, far outdistancing the $165.70 spent on "eye glasses, braces, etc." On the other hand, there was now a radiographic

department busy X-raying patients at a cost of $600 in salaries
and $1,821.01 in supplies. The laboratories were quite magnifi-
cently supported. Salaries and wages there amounted to
$7,874.25, outdistancing the salaries and wages paid for house-
keeping, laundry, or cleaning. At the Country Sanitarium, the
farm was still running at a loss, "Excess of Farm Expenses over
Farm Revenue" amounting to more than $4,000.

Apart from the city subsidy to the institution, there was little
municipal or state aid for the poor or disabled. The Social Service Department at Montefiore tried to do as much as possible
for patients and families without official help. In 1915, Miss
Hallahan, the first professional social service worker, resigned
and was replaced by Mollie Smith, a former member of the
Mount Sinai social welfare staff. Smith took a broad view of the
lives of the poor: "Poverty is a many-sided thing . . . related to
the physical, mental and moral state of the individual and the
environmental conditions in our Social and Economic Life." She
was assisted by "a volunteer Committee of ten women
(Auxiliary Members) who meet semi-monthly for the purpose
of discussing the family problems of our patients." The Social
Service Department was actually an activity of the Auxiliary,
now headed by Mrs. Simon Borg's daughter-in-law, Mrs. Sidney
Borg. The department met many needs: "five patients supplied
with abdominal binders, three with eye-glasses, and five given
free dental treatment, two receiving entire sets of teeth. Clothing was supplied to forty patients. Fifteen families were supplied with coal last winter."

During her first year, Miss Smith and her committee "cared
for 528 cases . . . and paid 1,700 visits of investigation, cooperation and advice." For several years after that the records show
frequent changes in the name of the paid worker, until in the
twenties another Miss Smith, Minnie, achieved informal tenure
in the position.

No patients were discharged until their homes were visited
and evaluated. Employment was found for some discharged
patients, and for those who could not work arrangements were
made with a "Charity Organization" to help the family.

In 1917 the Social Service Department began working with the children who were patients. Applicants were visited at home, and families of children who were already patients interviewed. A special effort was made to find out what had happened to ex-patients. "All the children that have been discharged from our Institution since January 1915 were followed up and it was found that many of them were without supervision and medical care. Some were in need of Institutional care, others of clinic supervision. For this purpose our Department has established an After-Care Clinic, where these children are examined periodically, and the mothers are advised how to guard against possible relapses. This clinic is of great service, especially to our discharged cardiac children who are kept under constant supervision. For the year there were 50 children under the observation of our clinic."

The Auxiliary, as well as setting up and helping to run the Social Service Department, provided many other services to the patients. No longer able to keep up with the sewing and mending of all the linens and clothing, they oversaw the purchase of these items for the Home and kept a close eye on the quality of the housekeeping, running white-gloved fingers over areas likely to collect dust. Children were their special concern, and for many years they supplied both their entertainment and their education. With the move to the Bronx, arrangements were made for the New York City Board of Education to supply a teacher, and the Montefiore classroom became part of the public school system. The children officially graduated from elementary school, after which their room was regarded as an annex of the Evander Childs High School.

Almost from the beginning, the Auxiliary encouraged handicrafts to occupy the patients, and by 1916 there was a large "manual training program," the type of work severely segregated by sex. Two hundred women embroidered and crocheted. Fifty-six girls embroidered, sewed, and knitted as well as making flowers and baskets from raffia. Forty-eight men were taught basket weaving (not with raffia), chair caning, the making of bed netting, woodwork, waxwork, and clay modeling, while forty boys learned to make animal toys and weave mats. In 1918, these activities became the nucleus of a professional department, and Susan C. Johnson was hired as "Director of Occupations." During the first year, she was assisted by 150 students from the Teachers College of Columbia University. By the next year, the number of students had decreased to fourteen, public enthusiasm for occupational therapy apparently having been a side effect of the war.

This was a program that always had several aims in view: exercise for muscles weakened by illness, diversion for the patient, the development of skills that could be used to earn a living, and even, occasionally, the production of profits for the institution by sale of the items manufactured by the patients.

At first the activities were much the same as had been carried on in the manual training classes, but Johnson quickly realized that many of the patients, especially those at Bedford, would return to the world and could be given skills that would help them make a living. She pressed for a print shop and commercial and academic classes at Bedford as well as "better coordination between the placement of patients after discharge and the selection of their occupation while in the institution." She even set up a bee-keeping program at the Sanitarium, an occupation probably difficult for discharged patients to pursue if they returned to New York City.

Johnson's awareness of the patients' needs led her to think at length about the question of payment for their work. Recognizing that there were many levels of ability and different attitudes among the patients, she nevertheless felt that "the sale of the products of occupation to the institution or to the public is . . . the only rational means of disposal of such products, and . . . sales in themselves have considerable therapeutic value," since they proved to the patients the worth of their work.

Johnson's concern about money led her to reveal aspects of life at Montefiore usually not discussed in the written record. The patients were poor and so were the people responsible for their care. Hospital workers were traditionally paid low wages. The jobs attracted the least skilled newcomers to the city. "Tips" from patients were always illegal. In practice, they were given and accepted. However small, they were an important addition to the pittance earned by an orderly or porter. A tip could ensure speedy delivery of a bedpan—or one that had been warmed. Johnson, in her eagerness to prove the enthusiasm of the patients for occupational therapy, wrote: "When patients were first transferred to the Schiff Pavilion and before regular provision for transportation to the workshop in the main building was made, several of the patients who had been accustomed to coming to the workshops took the initiative and themselves secured the services of an orderly to transport them across the road and voluntarily remunerated him from their own small store."

Boredom made patients restless, and the Auxiliary, together with the young, unmarried women of the Social Welfare League, provided concerts, movies, and outings. Children were taken to the circus, and adults who could travel, on bus excursions. They ran a large library for patients. The Hebrew Orphan Asylum Band was glad to entertain. The patients from the South Pavilion, devoted to tuberculosis, could not attend the concerts in the dining hall because of the fear of infection, but they were presented with a victrola.

Almost as soon as the patients were settled into the long wards on Gun Hill Road, plans were made for expansion. The Trustees decided to capitalize on the growing acceptance of hospital care by the upper and middle classes by building a pavilion for private patients on the opposite side of Bainbridge Avenue from the existing hospital buildings.

Four of the Trustees donated the building funds and made up the difference when the cost exceeded the original estimate of $200,000 by $48,966.15. Schiff announced, rather mysteriously, that "the name of the Private Pavilion has, for reasons which strongly commended themselves to the Director, been changed to 'Van Cortlandt Private Hospital.' " Presumably, this was to prevent the venture from becoming too closely connected in the public mind with Montefiore's charitable care of the incurable. The Medical Board objected to the change of name. The Trustees, hoping to attract about a hundred private patients, decided that any profits would be used to subsidize the regular work of the Hospital and they thought carefully about its management. A separate application form was devised for the use of private patients. Those physicians who donated their time to Montefiore and graduates of the house staff training program were to be given the privilege of admitting private patients. Other physicians, not connected with Montefiore, would have to hand over the care of their patients in the private pavilion to a Montefiore doctor.

Three kinds of patients were not to be admitted: "patients with contagious diseases," "insane, demented and idiotic patients," and "tuberculous patients." Apparently a distinction had to be made between tuberculosis and other contagious diseases.

At first a suggestion was made that a married doctor be hired to run the private pavilion so that his wife could act as head nurse and matron, but the decision was later made for the "pavilion to have a Resident Physician and a Head Nurse, the latter to act also as matron." (Montefiore always seems to have used "matron" to mean housekeeper and not, as in English usage, supervising nurse.)

The few semiprivate patients in the main building were charged $20 a week. The fees suggested for private patients were: "room without bath, $35 per week; room with bath, $45 per week; suite of rooms, $75 per week." Special nurses and special orderlies would cost $20 a week. Payments were to be made in advance, and one week's notice of departure was required. All wheelchairs, dressings, and drugs, except Salvarsan (used in treatment of syphilis), were included in the room charges. All special beverages, orthopedic appliances, X-ray examinations, and all special chemical and pathological tests cost extra. There would be a $5 charge for the use of the operating room. The Medical Board was concerned that these fees might be too high for middle-class patients, and the Board of Trustees agreed to reconsider the matter.

Before the pavilion could be fully tested, however, world events intervened. The nineteen acres of land on the north-eastern corner of Gun Hill Road and Bainbridge Avenue, directly opposite the Van Cortlandt Private Hospital, belonged to Columbia University. The grounds, known as the Columbia Oval, contained a clubhouse, a grandstand, tennis courts, and a running track. When the United States entered World War I in 1917, the Oval was taken over by the government and covered with barracks-like buildings to become part of United States Army General Hospital No. 1. The Trustees turned over their brand-new private hospital to the Army for the accommodation of the officers.

The war affected the institution in other ways. A Red Cross Auxiliary was organized by Mrs. Robert Isaac of the Ladies' Auxiliary. The group met at Mrs. Isaac's Portchester residence all during the summer to cut materials for surgical dressings. Back at the Home, the patients were involved in rolling bandages and knitting socks and balaclavas for the men at the front. Many of the younger members of the house and attending staffs enlisted. Some of the Trustees—Harold M. Lehman, Walter E. Meyer, Louis J. Robertson, and Fred Stein—went to Washington to help run the wartime government. Schiff acknowledged that the prosperity that war brought to the country had had an effect on public health: "Owing to war conditions, and in particular, to the highly remunerative work which was so readily obtainable, applications, especially at the Country Sanitarium, diminished somewhat." And Schiff, on the advice of his daughter Frieda, gave up speaking German in public.

CHAPTER

7

A New Order

Nineteen-twenty brought the end of an era. That summer, Jacob Schiff, seventy-three years old, was not feeling well. His doctor suggested that, instead of Bar Harbor, he try a higher altitude at Dixville Notch in New Hampshire, from where Schiff wrote to his friends complaining that he was not able to take his usual strenuous hikes. When the family went to Sea Bright in New Jersey for the later summer, he still was not fit but insisted on fasting for Yom Kippur. The next day, he returned to the Fifth Avenue mansion, where he died on September 25.

A world without Jacob Schiff seemed unthinkable. The minutes of the meeting of the Board of Trustees at which his colleagues, in a state of shock, made arrangements for memorial services did not mention him by name. The story in *The Montefiore Echo* was headlined "Our 'Little Father' Passes On." The death was a front-page story in the New York *Times*, the account of Schiff's life occupying the entire second page. The rich and the famous attended the services at Temple Emanu-El. Thousands and thousands of the poor and unknown lined Fifth

Avenue and the whole route of the cortege, following Schiff to his grave. Montefiore Home and Hospital was officially represented at the funeral by Dr. Wachsmann, Mr. Goodman, and Dr. Gabel, the rabbi.

The Succoth services at the Home, held October 4, became a memorial. The synagogue was draped in "the somber tones of mourning." The *Echo* reported that "Dr. Gabel, in English, delivered a stirring eulogy of our great benefactor, moving many of the congregation to tears." Another memorial service was held at Montefiore on November 4. According to the *Echo*: "Those present included directors, directresses, attending physicians, administrative officials, and a representation of patients, besides, of course, the immediate family of Mr. Schiff." The patients collected $219.65 to pay for a bronze memorial tablet.

In that same year, another link to the past was broken with the death of Simon Baruch at the age of eighty-one, soon after the publication of his last book, still preaching hydrotherapy and subsidized by his son Bernard. At Montefiore, the new President of the Board of Trustees, S. G. Rosenbaum, was eloquent about Baruch: "In stately appearance and in charm of manner he exemplified the finest type of dignified and courteous Southern gentleman and physician."

The two deaths symbolized the end of the old ways at the Hospital. The President of the Board of Trustees could no longer dominate the institution as the sole source of power, not only because there would not be another with the wealth and personality of Jacob Schiff, but even more because no layman could ever again presume to direct medical affairs. There had been a vast increase in medical knowledge since the founding of Montefiore. From this time forward, power would be shared between the Trustees and the physicians. The increase in medical knowledge was matched by the agreement of doctors upon the acceptance of that knowledge as a common professional belief, with which no lay Trustees could confidently argue. Dr. David Marine, the discoverer of the iodine treatment for goiter, came to Montefiore as Chief of Pathology, the effectiveness of his iodized salt not a matter of opinion but accepted as scientifically proven, as were the diagnostic power of X-rays and the necessary sterility of operating rooms.

Montefiore and the world were different places: Jacob Schiff and Simon Baruch and Tsar Nicholas were all dead; the flood stream of immigration was stopped, dammed up by restrictive legislation. World War I and the influenza epidemic of 1917 left behind a flotsam of survivors needing long-term care in a Montefiore that attempted to establish credibility as a twentieth-century scientific institution by eliminating the word "Home" from its title, becoming "The Montefiore Hospital for Chronic Diseases."

As if in recognition of a new order, Siegfried Wachsmann resigned. The man who succeeded him as Director also came from a German Jewish background. He was a young, enthusiastic proponent of the new scientific medicine, an idealist about society and about health care. As a physician, Ernst Boas showed profound concern for his patients, but he also worried about all who were poor, or sick, or suffered discrimination. He lived a more than full professional life as a physician in private practice, a researcher, an administrator, and an agitator for public health causes, constantly questioning his own achievements, never able to feel that he had reached the high standards he set for himself and others, never feeling that he could reach the standard set by his father.

His father, Franz Boas, became the first professor of anthropology at Columbia University, a post he held for thirty-seven years. His monumental energy was used to promulgate a new viewpoint for the scientific study of the human race. Traditional anthropology was strongly influenced in the nineteenth century both by the inappropriate biological model of Darwinism and by the common tendency in Europeans to see themselves as superior to the rest of the human race. Boas was not impressed with this competitive and ethnocentric view of social achievement. He saw all people as struggling with the same problems in living together and coming up with different family and community solutions, all societies as equally valuable and worthy of respectful study. His son was to inherit this egalitarian point of view.

Ernst Philip Boas was born in 1891 in Worcester, Massachusetts, while his father was still teaching at Clark. He grew up speaking both German and English and all his life was a prolific composer of letters in two languages. After completing his undergraduate studies at Columbia, he stayed on as a medical student.

To his father he wrote of his problems in getting practical experience in those days when a physician's education took place largely in the lecture hall. "I tried to get into a medical clinic but the man whom I had to see was never there. One day I met one of the anatomy teachers, and he asked me whether I would care to work in the surgery clinic. I agreed to do this." In these pre-antibiotic days, infection of wounds was the commonest of occurrences, with attempts made to keep patients with infected wounds away from the uninfected. Ernst was assigned to the "pus section." At the clinic he learned something about class and medicine, and the use of the poor as teaching material: "Yesterday I almost cut an abscess. My hands were aseptic and the doctor was giving me the cocaine needle for injection, when he discovered that the patient was an employee of the clinic. So then he performed the operation. Apparently only outside patients are put in our hands—the poor things."

In 1914, after receiving his M.D., he encountered considerable difficulty in securing an internship, being turned down by four hospitals before being accepted at Mount Sinai. The reasons for his difficult search are not obscure. Jacob Schiff's fears about the impact of large-scale Jewish immigration had been realized, with anti-Semitism virulent, widespread, and officially sanctioned. In the late nineties, Jacob Schiff had written to Bishop Potter of New York complaining of "the spirit which, as by a tacit understanding, excludes the Hebrews from the Trustee-room of Columbia College, of the public museums, the public library, and many similar institutions." The widespread discrimination that existed in education affected the lives of thousands of young men and women. Sororities, fraternities, honor societies, and eating clubs in colleges, large and small, excluded Jews. Professional schools established quotas that kept out all but a small proportion of Jews. Columbia University set up regional quotas, and since most Jews lived in the Eastern cities, their numbers were cut back.

After a brief period in private practice, when he did a little pathology at Montefiore, Boas joined the Army and served in France. Beginning to worry about making a living after the war, he wrote to his father: "I wrote to Dr. Wachsmann at Montefiore the other day in regard to getting connected with his hospital again when I get back . . . although I hope to be out of debt when I leave the Army, I'll have to borrow again to start in practice." Back in New York, he began building up a practice, but by the spring of the next year his life was changed. He was a father and the Director of Montefiore. With the job came the twelve-room house on 210th Street formerly occupied by Dr. Wachsmann.

President Rosenbaum announced that the Trustees believed that "in the selection of Dr. Boas they have chosen a man who will uphold the best traditions of the Hospital." Boas was to preside over an era that looked more steadily to the future than to the past. He had great plans for the hospital and great hopes for their fulfillment: "I am putting thru a complete reorganization of the professional services, and hope that we will really get somewhere. Up to the present [May 1921] I have had no time for medical work, but I did not expect that for the first few months. In another month I expect to start on the heart wards. I really think that things will turn out very well for me. But I must always be on guard not to get tied up too much with the administrative end. I think that will be easy when we are organized. Up to now I have gotten along very well with the directors [the Board] which after all is very important."

His feelings about his ability to make changes at the hospital varied: "I have my ups and downs. Some days I am very discouraged, and on others I am very optimistic."

That summer he wrote to his parents: "Friday, Dr. Marine, our director of laboratories, had dinner with us and went downtown with me to the meeting of the Executive Committee of the Medical Board. The meeting was very disappointing. Only two of the members understand what it is all about and others always wish to make compromises which are ineffectual. It is a little difficult for me because I am so young and many of the doctors present have been my teachers. Now I have to tell them how to run their sections."

That this meeting was held "downtown" indicated one of Montefiore's basic problems. Most of the attending physicians who made up the Medical Board, including all the chiefs of sections (except Marine in Pathology), practiced in Manhattan. Mount Sinai was the hospital in which they were chiefly interested and to which they admitted most of their paying patients. Their interest in Montefiore was charitable or scientific. Visiting the hospital on the outskirts of the Bronx was time-consuming. The subway did not yet come to the end of Jerome Avenue. A walk from the last subway stop was long and filled with the hazards provided by the goats which roamed the neighborhood. A trip by automobile took considerable time in a world not only without expressways but, in the area around Montefiore, without paved roads. The physicians could not put in the time needed to build up efficient departments, to visit patients, or to supervise house staff.

Boas had the optimism and arrogance of youth, prepared to take on these giants from Manhattan, writing to his father: "Elsberg especially causes many difficulties. There is nothing we can do with him and I am afraid we shall simply have to get rid of him." This was Charles Elsberg, one of the most famous neurosurgeons of the day. Boas was also willing to tackle the great B. S. Oppenheimer, now the Chief of Medicine, who, according to the young Director, "has no push and will accomplish nothing by himself."

The Board backed their choice. Before the end of the year, Boas was reporting: "The Directors are remarkably generous and tractable. I have been able to put through all of my plans to date, although they are already costing the hospital about $50,000 more a year. I really believe that in a few years Montefiore will be known as a scientific hospital of the first water."

Boas had no experience or training in the administration of a large and complex institution. He had, however, firm views on the social and medical treatment of patients and on the direction in which medicine should be moving. Still busy improving his knowledge of cardiology, the specialty he had chosen, he saw specialization, as he had in his days at Mount Sinai, as the wave of the future. He believed that, as a natural corollary of the growth of medical science, no one person could fully command all the knowledge available and that physicians must concentrate on particular areas of medicine.

Once that was agreed upon, drawing up the dividing lines was difficult. Formal organization developed slowly, piecemeal, and from a variety of roots. The very act of division produced questions that have never been fully or satisfactorily answered. Should specialties follow parts of the body, as in cardiology? Diseases, as in oncology? Or the service rendered, as in surgery? When Boas took over at Montefiore, few of these problems had been worked out on a national level. The only specialty board which conducted examinations was that in ophthalmology. Boas was free to carve out the divisions of his hospital as he saw fit, providing, of course, that the professional staff agreed with him. He more or less followed the categories into which the patients seemed to fall, setting up Divisions of Medicine, Neurology, Tuberculosis, Cancer, Laboratories, and Surgery. There was only one subdivision under Medicine—the Dermatological Service—and none under any of the others except Surgery, which included General Surgical, Orthopedic, Laryngological, Ophthalmological, Neurosurgical, and Gynecological Services. The most unusual division was the Cancer Division, quite possibly the only one in the United States at the time. Few general hospitals had the number of beds devoted to cancer that there were at Montefiore. The separate division actually lasted only two years until the Chief, Dr. I. Levin, left to go to the Rockefeller Institute and the Cancer Division became part of the Surgical Division. Two services, Dentistry and Roentgenology (X-rays), were not formally attached to any division.

Boas reorganized and strengthened the house staff. Before his arrival these people were designated as "assistant physicians," with one of the number the "house physician." Eight of them, plus a dentist and a druggist, served the patients in the Bronx, while two were assigned to Bedford. Boas' house staff, at the end of his first full year of service, consisted of eight "resident physicians"—one each assigned to the Medical, Neurological, Surgical, Tuberculosis, and Cancer Services and the Private Pavilion, and two to the Bedford Sanitarium—ten "internes," and a druggist. There was also a dental intern who assisted the dentist, who came in four half-days a week. By the time Boas left, in 1928, there were over forty interns, externs, and residents on the wards, attracted by the growing scientific stature of the place and kept busy by the intensive patient care and research upon which Boas insisted. And every year, at a time when 95 percent of the hospitals in the United States refused to take female house staff, three or four women appeared on the roster.

Boas pointed out to the Board the difficulties of attracting a good medical staff of doctors willing to volunteer their time to Montefiore: "General hospitals have little difficulty in recruiting their medical staffs. Usually the applicants for appointment are so numerous that a good selection can be made, and a high degree of efficiency demanded. Physicians seek hospital appointments because the appointment gives them some prestige, and affords them an opportunity of placing their private patients in the public or private wards where they can study them to the best advantage. The privilege of treating private patients in the institution contributes an important item to their income. And finally and most importantly their work in the hospital affords unexcelled opportunities for gaining clinical experience on a very large scale. The average length of stay of a patient in most general hospitals is about two weeks. Thus a physician who is in charge of a ward service of thirty beds will see 650 patients during the year, allowing for an average bed occupancy of eighty-five per cent."

At the most, a physician at Montefiore in the same position would see 90 patients. Additionally, the physician in a chronic disease hospital saw little change in the condition of his patients. "Finally, certain types of patients found in a chronic hospital are disagreeable to examine, they may be incontinent and dirty, or they may be perpetual complainers."

He suggested measures to make service at Montefiore more

attractive: each attending physician should have charge of a larger number of patients to make for greater variety and the assistance of a junior physician or resident to help with the workload; adequate resources for complete diagnosis and investigation; and good research facilities.

At the same time, Boas was functioning as a physician, visiting patients on the wards, working on his research in cardiology, and campaigning in the outside world on behalf of the needs of the chronically ill, most of whom were not receiving the kind of care provided at Montefiore. He saw long-term illness as one of the great social problems of the day. Most of the nation's long-term illness was treated or, more truthfully, neglected—not in institutions like Montefiore—but either in the patients' own homes or in those public places known as poorhouses, workhouses, or almshouses, where medical or nursing care was limited or nonexistent.

At Montefiore the annual meeting of 1923 looked briefly to the past—but then leaped ahead with news of the exciting scientific present. The headlines in the city newspapers the next day read: "Insulin Saves Lives at Montefiore Home." The New York *Times* was the only newspaper in town to have a reasonably accurate story and even then did not acknowledge Montefiore's new status as a hospital. The other papers had more sensational headlines: "Diabetes Serum Complete Cure." "All Doctors to Get Diabetes Cure Soon." "New Cure Ends Diabetes Curse, Asserts Flexner."

Some of the statements actually made at the meeting were as inaccurate as the headlines. The Flexner brother who spoke was Simon, head of the Rockefeller Institute. He declared that the discovery of insulin was accidental, a statement that would have amazed the discoverers, the Canadians Frederick Banting and Charles Best, who had known exactly what they were looking for. The speedy involvement of the Rockefeller Institute was more dependent on accident. Frederick Taylor Gates, a Baptist clergyman who, after a successful campaign to raise funds for the founding of the University of Chicago, became an assistant and adviser to John D. Rockefeller, was, like his wife, diabetic.

He read an early story about insulin in a Canadian newspaper and wrote to suggest that some of the substance be obtained. Rockefeller complied, and the small supply that arrived was tested on Mr. and Mrs. Gates. The next letter to Rockefeller expressed their euphoria at their improved state. He urged Rockefeller to become involved. In collaboration with the Institute and the group in Toronto, six hospitals in the New York area were chosen, Montefiore among them because of Dr. A. I. Ringer's active research program in diabetes.

By the fall of 1922, the Metabolic Service at Montefiore was reorganized, a special ward set aside, and extra nurses employed. Ringer was given special laboratory facilities and the services of a chemist. He himself contributed $600 to be used for a yearly fellowship in metabolism so that he could have a second assistant. Eighty patients were treated, and the audience at the annual meeting was regaled with stories of triumphs. Five of the patients were already in diabetic coma before help arrived and they were revived by insulin. Ringer reported that only a few days before a twenty-three-year-old man had been brought to the hospital in the last stages of the disease. After three injections of insulin he was sitting up in bed reading a magazine. A fifty-year-old man who had been pronounced incurable was now on his way to Europe.

The institution had long been concerned with the medical and social futures of discharged tubercular patients. In 1920, more than half of those admitted with the early signs of tuberculosis were sent home able to resume their former occupations or take up some lighter form of work. In that same year, a clinic for sufferers from heart disease was opened. Dr. M. W. Goldstein was the Director. Most of the patients were children.

By the next year, space had been set aside in the East Building basement for a clinic that was open every Saturday afternoon. Of the fifteen patients, some were former inpatients, some came from the neighborhood, and some were from the cardiac class at Public School No. 4. The public schools of the day took their public health roles very seriously and many had special classes set aside for children with physical problems.

By the next year, there was a Cancer Clinic, where out-patients received X-ray and radium treatment. Diabetic and Physiotherapy Clinics followed. At the same time, the physicians were making house calls on former patients when they were unable to visit the clinics.

Radium and X-rays had been used in treatment at Montefiore since before the war, but in 1924 a separate "Radiotherapeutic Service" was set up under Dr. Maurice Lenz.

Two and a half million dollars' worth of construction took place under Boas and Samuel Sachs, Chairman of the Building Committee of the Board: the new nurses' residence and the total rebuilding of the Country Sanitarium. The old wooden units at Bedford had been deliberately designed to provide a maximum of fresh air and a minimum of privacy, at a time when exercise was seen as a necessary part of treatment. Now the opposite was viewed as essential to the healing process and the new buildings were planned to provide "rest, comfort, mental relaxation, pleasant and cheerful surroundings inside and outside of the buildings as well as . . . active treatment for pulmonary tuberculosis and its complications." Provision was made for 220 patients, those who were totally bedridden and those who, after treatment, improved to the extent that they became "ambulant." Fresh air still held a magic fascination: transoms and wide-opening windows provided for gusts of it at all times, and the colder, the better. The wards where the ambulant and semi-ambulant patients lived were kept at 50° F. in the winter.

CHAPTER

8

The Doctors

B oas' endeavor to make Montefiore a respectable scientific institution was greatly aided by the arrival of one of the great scientists of the twentieth century. For twenty-five years, from 1920 to 1945, the laboratories at Montefiore were headed by a man remarkable on many counts. David Marine was world-famous for his discovery of an effective therapy for goiter, and distinguished in medical circles for his assiduous exploration of the thyroid gland and the endocrine system preceding and succeeding that discovery. The first full-time chief at the Hospital, he was Protestant at a time when almost the entire medical staff and almost all the patients were Jewish.

Marine's own greatest accomplishment was to be not in the cure but in the prevention of one of the diseases that had plagued whole populations from the time when human beings first spread out from their original homes. Upon graduation from Johns Hopkins he accepted a position as resident pathologist at Lakeside Hospital, part of Western Reserve University in Cleveland.

From 1917 to 1920, Marine carried out a successful large-scale goiter-prevention campaign with the girls in the fifth to the twelfth grade in the Akron public schools. Almost half of the girls had a slight goiter. A political storm broke out over the Akron experiment as an invasion of personal rights, and it was in Michigan that the first follow-up took place.

In the meantime, in 1920, Marine moved to Montefiore. In the course of arranging for his appointment, Marine met Jacob Schiff. "In a ten-minute meeting regarding the reorganization and expansion of the laboratory facilities I pointed out that it would be desirable to purchase complete sets of the important scientific journals, which would entail possibly a $5,000 outlay during the next two years. Mr. Schiff had apparently made his decision before I had finished the statement, for at once he said, 'That can be done. What next?'"

The salary of the new Director of Laboratories was set at $8,000. Marine spent much of his first year at Montefiore organizing the Division of Laboratories. He had a full-time staff of seventeen people divided among Departments of Physiology, Chemistry, and Pathology and a combined Department of Bacteriology and Serology. In addition, he had three voluntary assistants working on special problems. He also set up Ward Laboratories in each of the clinical divisions under the jurisdiction of the chiefs of those divisions to take care of the tests for patients, and thus the staff of the main laboratory could devote all their time to research in the "general field of internal secretions and their interrelations." Marine added: "All the Departments have been actively engaged on problems correlated with this general subject." His labs occupied the third floor of the West Building and his animals were housed on the flat roof above. The library was rapidly expanded with 903 volumes of medical journals and 90 books added during the year. A workshop equipped with "a lathe, drill press and other wood and metal working tools was part of the complex."

By the next year, Marine was complaining: "The Laboratory is already overcrowded. Additional space for stacks and reading rooms is urgently needed for our growing library. A new building for research will soon be necessary if we are to retain our leadership in the field of research medicine with which we are now prominently identified. . . . The greatly increased demand for metabolic rate determinations illustrates the interest and increasing importance of this diagnostic measure." He might well have added that the increase in the use of laboratory testing of all kinds reflected the increasingly scientific orientation of medicine at Montefiore.

Around Boas gathered a group of young cardiologists who developed their own private practices while continuing their inquiry and study at the Hospital and remained a part of Montefiore for as long as fifty years: Harry Gross, Abe Jezer, Leonard Tarr, and John Schwedel.

Geza Nemet was also part of that long tradition of political refugees who found a haven at Montefiore. Born in Hungary, a graduate of the medical school of the University of Budapest, he served his internship in Frankfurt, Germany. He was on the medical faculty in Frankfurt and at the University of Berlin, but returned to Hungary to take part in the revolution led by Béla Kun. When that was suppressed by Admiral Horthy, Nemet fled to the United States and Montefiore, where he worked as an attending physician and chief of the adult cardiac clinic.

One of the greatest of the band of brilliant cardiologists was invited to come to Gun Hill Road by Boas before he became Director. Pincus Schwartz spent his early childhood in Bucharest, and came to the United States with his father at the age of ten. He received his M.D. from the College of Physicians and Surgeons in 1922 and interned at Fordham Hospital. It was the chief of service at Fordham who introduced him to Ernst Boas. "At that time," Schwartz recalled, "Montefiore had no interns and Boas asked me to work for the private pavilion for a couple of months . . . Then I came into the hospital proper as an intern, and I became a resident physician under Oppenheimer, and here I remained ever since."

Boas and Schwartz became good friends, the younger man staying in Boas' house, enjoying and guarding the library when the Director went to Wilton for the summer. Their feelings about each other were always warm. Schwartz's emotions about

B. S. Oppenheimer ran a wider gamut: "He was a hard task-master. I was house physician. He would have me write papers and put his name on them without giving me credit. One time I had a severe hemorrhage from the lung and he sent his secretary out for me to dictate the paper. I was too sick. He read it at the Academy and didn't give me credit. Then I just went up in the air and I minced no words. I called him a bearded bastard in front of everybody else and I told him I had no use for him. [Despite this] we became very good friends."

For fifteen years, Schwartz was in charge of the children's cardiac clinic, a post that necessitated working closely with the members of the Ladies' Auxiliary, who regarded the children as their special charge. They could be both generous and, from the physician's point of view, difficult: "I worked in the children's cardiac clinic with Mrs. Stroock. We got along very well but I couldn't tolerate some of her demands. It was too much for me, but she was a very generous person. . . . We had a very large children's cardiac clinic, well over 600 children. It was one of the largest in the country, and it was a very popular clinic."

Other young doctors were attracted by the reputation of the Division of Neurology. In 1920, 424 people were treated at Montefiore for "diseases of the nervous system." The one patient who left "cured" suffered from Sydenham's chorea (also called St. Vitus's dance), a condition in which the patient makes quick, uncontrollable movements. Thirty-eight neurological cases left improved, 99 left unimproved, 108 died, and 178 remained in the hospital. Eighteen could be considered psychiatric cases: sixteen with hysteria (fourteen of them women) and two (one of each sex) with manic-depressive psychosis.

Nineteenth-century physicians at Montefiore were aware of the difficulties of sorting out the vagaries of the nervous system and were willing to accept all the blockages of neural communication as of equal interest whatever their origin; they admitted the old man paralyzed as a result of a stroke and the young girl whose hysteria prevented her from moving her arm. They treated both. As late as 1915, the record shows that two patients suffering from "neurosis" were discharged "improved." Gradually, however, Montefiore adopted the practice of most general hospitals and stopped admitting those with purely psychiatric conditions.

When Boas set up his system of clinical divisions at Montefiore he did not include psychiatry. Some of the leading neurologists at Montefiore were actively hostile to the Freudian theories then crossing the Atlantic. Bernard Sachs was given to public derision, and the understanding of psychoanalytic theory on the part of other members of the staff of the Division of Neurology appears to have been somewhat limited.

The basic link between psychiatry and neurology remained, however. In 1934, the American Board of Psychiatry and Neurology was established to conduct examinations and set standards in both disciplines, and many of the people who trained in the Division of Neurology at Montefiore went on to practice psychiatry.

This large, active program in teaching, research, and patient care in neurology was remarkable in the world of medicine in the 1920s. In addition to those whose central nervous systems had been injured or attacked directly, there were all those whose condition was caused by syphilis or tuberculosis or typhoid fever or smallpox—all the infectious diseases that still raged through the land. Most of the sufferers received little or no medical care. The situation had changed little, if at all, since 1910 when an article in the *Journal of the American Medical Association* declared: "In all America there is scarcely a general hospital with neurologic wards worthy of the name . . ."

Until 1928, Harvard, Columbia (which used Montefiore as its teaching hospital), and the University of Pennsylvania were the only medical schools in the United States with departments of neurology.

Within this context, the Division of Neurology at Montefiore was enormous and the number of physicians who trained there was extraordinary. One hundred and fifty beds were normally occupied by neurology cases and a large number of beds in the Schiff Pavilion (where the patients received only custodial care) were occupied by people with neurological conditions.

The patients were highly valued as teaching material. "Museum" was a word frequently used to describe the collection of suffering deformities. Neurology was the division that had the most active teaching program with Columbia. The students came up each year to look at the museum specimens, who, in turn, grew quite knowledgeable about their own symptoms. One long-term victim of multiple sclerosis was exhibited to the students so often that on occasion he would prompt the instructor with a remark such as "Pro-fes-sor, you-forgot-to-tell-them that-I'm-euphoric," in the scanning, rhythmical speech that is one of the telltale signs of the illness.

Bernard Sachs, who did so much to foster neurology at Montefiore, looked like a professor. He inspired awed respect. Boas' Chief of Neurology, Simon Philip Goodhart, was different. His initials were rumored to stand for "Simon Pure." Boas' successor, E. M. Bluestone, described him as "my precious friend . . . endowed with a name which accurately described his character and warm personality. . . . He was short and spare, with a cocked head that seemed to rest on his chest as a sort of pedestal, with a look on his face that was always thoughtful and serious even when he was telling a witty anecdote. . . . Always shy, and perhaps consciously self-effacing."

The Board of Trustees, before appointing Boas, had actually urged Goodhart to give up his post as Chief to become Director of Montefiore. Perhaps it was his shyness that compelled him to decline and allowed Boas to take over.

Under the new regime there were rapid improvements in the organization of the division. In 1921, Abraham Rabiner was a clinical assistant in the Outpatient Department at Mount Sinai. Most of the Montefiore neurologists had appointments at Mount Sinai, and after a neurological conference at Mount Sinai, Rabiner had coffee with a group which included Israel Wechsler, Isadore Abrahamson, and Moses Keschner. They were dissatisfied with the situation at Montefiore, where there was no full-time resident working on the neurological wards, keeping track of the patients between the scattered visits these busy physicians were able to make to the Bronx. They offered the job to Rabiner. Rabiner thus became the first neurological resident at Montefiore and, beginning in January 1922, he set about reorganizing the service, arranging for regular teaching rounds and conferences. After a year and a half at Montefiore, he traveled to England and Germany for study and then came back to Montefiore to help set up the first neuropathological laboratory, of which Walter M. Kraus became the head.

His own specialty was the dyskinesias (conditions in which the power of voluntary movement is impaired), and he was quick to use the new technologies available for observation and teaching, recording the distinctive movements of his patients in motion pictures, which he showed at in-hospital and national conferences.

Neurology in the nineteenth century and the early twentieth century was concerned with sorting out and describing all the different conditions from which patients suffered, deciding what particular symptoms went together, what movements or lack of movements could be a basis for diagnosis. The awe-inspiring neurologists who walked the wards dazzled their students with the brilliance and speed of their judgments. Residents talked of Moses Keschner diagnosing from the movement of a big toe. The neuropathologist and the autopsy were immensely important because there frequently could not be a positive confirmation of the inspired guess until the dead body was explored for its secrets.

CHAPTER
9

Nursing

"A few were excellent but the large majority were shiftless, untruthful, independent and cruel to the patients. Scientific study was impossible when the doctors had to depend on the attendants for part of their data." Thus Mildred Constantine, the first Director of the Nursing School that Montefiore ran for ten years, from 1922 to 1932, described the undertrained, underpaid women who, before that period, provided most of the nursing care to the patients who spent months or even years at the Home for Chronic Diseases.

The establishment of the school was one of the early steps taken by Boas to upgrade the level of scientific and humanitarian concern. In selling the idea of the need for trained nurses, however, Constantine unconsciously revealed the most serious flaw in the structure of her profession: "We find repeatedly that one interested student replaces two attendants and one graduate nurse."

Trained nurses were as essential to the development of the modern hospital as physicians. Patients recover only if they are fed, bathed, bedpanned, and given the treatment and medication prescribed by the doctor. The roads traveled by the two professions were quite different. The training of a physician allowed him to become an independent businessman. If he attracted the right clientele, he himself could achieve considerable wealth. Hospitals and doctors developed relationships as convoluted as the general economics of medical care. In many hospitals, physicians wielded dominant power. In others, they shared power with administrators and trustees. As governments at various levels became involved in health care, physicians' organizations strongly influenced the terms on which the assistance was accepted.

No nurses' organization ever achieved the fearsome power of the American Medical Association in its heyday. Even when nursing schools escaped from hospitals to the groves of academe, they never achieved the prestige or the independent status of medical schools. Nurses rarely achieved power within American hospitals except in Catholic institutions, where nursing sisters were able to climb the administrative ladder. Very rarely could nurses go into business for themselves. They were almost always employees, seldom in a position to question the terms of their employment. The employment itself was insecure. Until after World War II, a majority of graduate nurses were employed, not in hospitals, but in private homes, usually badly paid, often treated as domestic servants, while the work in hospitals was done by unpaid students.

The two professions shared one feature: for at least the first half of the twentieth century, both doctors and nurses were expected to contribute their labor in return for education. Hospitals set up nursing schools whose students trained on the job and supplied the bulk of the patient care side by side with unpaid or poorly paid interns and residents. On the whole, nurses came from different social classes and ethnic groups than physicians. Nursing tended to attract working-class and lower-middle-class women, as a way to a profession for those who lacked the money to finance a college degree, the nursing schools providing board and lodging, often uniforms as well, and sometimes a small allowance. Every year enough nurses married doctors to keep alive the dream of upward mobility.

Ethnically, nurses and physicians tended to come from different groups. While medicine was always seen as a highly desirable way of life for Jewish males, Jewish females had to fight institutions and families as hard as their gentile sisters for entry to medical schools. There were religious taboos for Orthodox women, whether as nurses or doctors, participating in the physical care of men not members of their families, and as long as the only employment open to the graduate nurse was in private homes, where she barely outranked the cleaning woman, nursing was not likely to attract a group which had traditionally shunned domestic service.

In the twenties and thirties most of the nurses at Montefiore were Christian, and all were white. The Nursing School which opened at Montefiore Hospital for Chronic Diseases in 1922 advertised widely in women's magazines, and many of the replies were from women trapped by poverty in little Southern towns.

The opening of the school did not solve all the staffing problems. Nurses willing to work at night were particularly hard to attract. While in 1923 the Van Cortlandt Private Pavilion was entirely staffed by graduate nurses, the ward patients were cared for by a mix of graduates, undergraduates, pupils, attendants, orderlies, and ward maids. (The duties of the ward maids were to "make empty beds; give tub baths; feed patients; dress patients; assist in getting patients up in chairs; clean chairs, tables, beds, utility rooms, windowsills and washbasins; stack linen, clean linen rooms; clean patients' finger and toenails and comb their hair.")

Constantine remained wary of attendants, warning against allowing them to approach any but the simplest of cases: "because the attendant after watching a graduate do the catheterizations and administer medicines soon feels that she can do these things herself and either becomes discontented and leaves or persuades a doctor or nurse to allow her to demonstrate her ability. Once she has done this it is a temptation to a busy graduate nurse to allow her to continue this practice. . . . This is one of the chief reasons why we feel attendants should be allowed only to care for Class C cases." (Class C comprised those patients requiring the least intensive care.)

In 1921 a study at Mount Sinai Hospital showed that the average patient at that acute-care institution received four hours and forty-nine minutes of nursing care in twenty-four hours. Constantine found that, at Montefiore, the time ranged from a minimum of one hour and six minutes for a diabetic child to a maximum of six hours and twenty minutes for an incontinent patient with a spastic paralysis of the legs. The average time per patient was four hours and fourteen minutes.

A few years later Alice Otto, R.N., described the nursing service at Montefiore. Like Constantine, she felt that the nursing of long-term illness required special qualities: "A hospital that cares for such patients requires nurses who are sympathetic, intelligent, and experienced in their profession. Each nurse must know her special field. She must continue her studies and read on these particular subjects. Her patience must be endless, she must exercise tact and above all, be kindhearted. The mental health of the patients is one of the most important things for her to consider. The nurse must know just how to handle her patient, when to approach him, and how to encourage him when his spirits droop."

Otto felt the nurse should be a firm disciplinarian with patients: "Everything must be done to avoid exciting these patients. Some believe that various treatments and medication will help them and ask for these constantly. Other patients are likely to develop sympathetic ailments, e.g., if one patient develops a headache or vomits, he must be separated from the others by having the curtain drawn around his bed, if for no other reason than to prevent other patients from developing the same symptoms by suggestion. Some patients are even taught by the nurses to speak and others to read. They must be taught personal hygiene . . . Some of the patients are in a degenerative mental condition and are only contented when they are left alone, permitted to expectorate without restriction, or given the bedpan as often as twenty times during the night.

"Ventilation is an everlasting problem in every institution but is more acute in the hospital which cares for the chronically ill. Many patients are dyspneic; some are fresh-air fiends; others feel that they cannot stand fresh air and insist that the windows be kept closed. All groups have to be appeased. The nurse herself must often hold the thermometer in place and make certain that the patient is not malingering. Many cardiac patients are on restricted fluids and must therefore be watched carefully. These patients often go to the bathroom and drink water when they are not under the observation of a reliable attendant."

Many different kinds of insects made life unpleasant for the patients. Flies were ubiquitous: the Bronx at this time still contained working farms and horse-drawn delivery wagons lined the streets with droppings. The *Echo* constantly urged on its readers the duty of killing a quota of flies each day. Patients suffering from pemphigus (a disease characterized by large blisters on the skin and mucous membranes) were given a daily potassium permanganate bath, after which, Otto explained, "the affected areas have to be covered carefully with dressings, otherwise flies may have access to those parts."

At least one aspect of hospital routine that has always irritated and baffled patients was avoided at Montefiore: "The patients cannot have morning care before seven o'clock, as is the case in other hospitals where they remain only two and three weeks, because a patient cannot be awakened at 5 a.m. for several months at a time, or longer, merely to have his face washed. This means additional work for the day nurses."

The total health of patients was the responsibility of an institution where they stayed for months or years: "Oral hygiene is a factor to be considered in the nursing care of the chronically ill. The oral hygienist, while making rounds, instructs the nurses how to clean the patients' teeth properly, and each nurse in turn reports the patients who are in need of dental treatment."

Nurses spent a great deal of time moving patients from one location to another: "Whenever the weather permits patients must be placed on the porches in the sunshine. This breaks the monotony of the day and also tends to make the patients stronger. They also become much more cheerful when exposed to sunshine and fresh air. Each patient is well wrapped in blankets and provided with a flask of drinking water and a bell. The nurses must watch the patients who are on the porches to see that they are always comfortable and warm."

Nurses were also part of the research team. In these early days of insulin therapy, all was uncertainty. Effects, good or bad, were often unpredictable and little understood. The strength of each succeeding batch of insulin was variable. Patients were watched carefully, both for their own safety and to add to the general store of knowledge about the new treatment. "Diabetic patients who have their legs amputated frequently develop abscessed stumps which require careful nursing attention."

Insulin brought well-founded hope. Radium brought a much less certain light to cancer patients: "When a patient receives radium treatment, a tag is placed on the edge of his bed stating the hour when the radium should be removed. The patient, however, must be watched carefully, since he may develop a high temperature, in which case the doctor must be notified immediately, as the radium will undoubtedly have to be removed. Patients who receive radiotherapy may not be given a hot water bag, since heat is often contraindicated; neither should iodine be applied to the parts treated with radium."

The hope was slight. Death constantly hovered in the cancer ward: "The condition of these patients changes quickly, and one who was apparently in good condition just a few months before may suddenly pass away. A patient with sarcoma at the base of the neck must be handled most carefully, since a fracture of the bone is likely to occur and thus precipitate death."

Some relief of pain and avoidance of secondary infection was all that could be given to most of these people: "Bedsores must be prevented since the tissues tend to break down easily. Enemas and vaginal douches are very painful and the nurse must be patient and kind. These patients become chilled very readily. Many hot water bags have to be used, but the temperature of the water must be carefully tested, since these patients are very sensitive to heat. Especially good technic must be used in giving hypodermic injections. Many patients have injections every three or four hours for many months; their extremities as a result are easily abscessed. Other infections also develop, as the vitality and resistance of these patients are very low."

The importance of nutrition and, interestingly enough, of vitamin C was recognized: "Cancer patients are placed on a high caloric diet and are advised to drink citrus fruit juices; it is therefore the nurse's duty to see that the patients receive them."

Heart patients were fed a diet of hope: "Chronic cardiac patients must be repeatedly assured that something is being done for them and that they are getting better."

Rest was the great therapy for cardiac patients, no excitement, no arguments. "The position of cardiac patients in bed is an important factor in their care. They must be propped up on pillows constantly and provided with a cardiac table, a reading table, or a food tray, on which a pillow is placed so that they can rest their arms and be comfortable. They find it easier to breathe when sitting up. They like to lean forward, therefore their arms, backs and heads must be supported."

The year 1925 was a notable one for the Nursing School. The first class of three graduated. By then the whole school consisted of fourteen students. (Numbers increased rapidly and soon each class numbered about twenty.) In that same year, the Board of Trustees finally acknowledged that the Van Cortlandt Private Pavilion would never attract enough paying patients to be worthwhile. The elegant building was converted into housing for the nurses, giving each graduate nurse her own room and attracting more nurses who were prepared to work the night shift.

Two years later, an eight-story annex was built at a cost of $385,000 to provide a Nurses Home with 110 beds, each in a separate room. By 1927 the 650 patients were cared for by 33 graduate nurses, 41 undergraduates, 76 pupils, 8 special nurses, 14 maids, and 37 orderlies.

The new Van Cortlandt Annex contained a large room suitable for dancing, and Constantine reported: "The house staff seem to enjoy this form of recreation. They have given several dances and have encouraged the nurses to give dances which they have attended in large numbers."

There were other gaieties: "The student nurses had a course of sightseeing which included visits to Museums, factories, and an ocean liner, lectures at the Metropolitan and Natural History Museums. The students' Sewing Circle has met once a week. . . . This is an informal gathering in the Instructor's rooms. The students mend, darn stockings, read aloud and discuss current events. It is not compulsory but has always been well attended."

Some services were provided to the nurses in residence. There were "electric irons" on each floor but no ironing was allowed in the rooms. Clean towels were issued on Tuesdays and Fridays if the soiled towels were left out "for the maid to exchange." Laundry was collected at 7 a.m. on Mondays.

Nurses were trained through a mix of lectures and practical experience on the wards, with the emphasis on the latter. The hours were long. Day nurses worked from 7 a.m. to 7 p.m., with two hours off a day and two afternoons a week beginning at 1 p.m.

A well-rounded nursing course required experience in an acute-care setting, and the students were sent for part of their time to Long Island College Hospital in Brooklyn Heights and to Bellevue, the largest and oldest of New York City's municipal hospitals.

CHAPTER
10
Patients, Invention, and Invective

Boas' relationship with patients was unlike that of any other administrator who was at Montefiore. Abraham Goldberg trained as an architect, his career halted when he became ill. Admitted to Montefiore at the age of thirty-eight, he died eleven years later. His life as a patient was active. From 1925 to 1934, he was the editor of *The Montefiore Echo*. Boas, anxious to involve those most concerned in the running of the institution, formed a Patient's Welfare Council and Goldberg became Chairman. Photographs show him in a three-piece suit with watch chain and tie, on the crutches on which he moved around the hospital.

Boas invited him to write the section on "Welfare and Entertainment" for his book. Goldberg began with a description of what was probably his own state of mind when he came to Montefiore: "To say that the realization of being classed with the chronic sick causes a mental cataclysm is to put it mildly. Reason is temporarily obliterated. Most such sufferers have a long history of seeking for a cure, and to many, an institution for the chronic represents the inevitable or final step, perhaps the end. These, then, are battered psychic victims laboring under the depressing anticipation of a future of unrelieved monotony and tedium."

He explained his need for vest and watch chain: "Permission to wear his own clothes and not a standard uniform is the first point of consideration which helps the patient maintain his equilibrium. Then, of course, there is the treatment to which he is subjected in respect to the worth of his personal dignity. Treated like an inferior, he would certainly feel inferior. On the other hand, permitting him to feel a sense of freedom is the beginning of self-confidence."

Both Boas and Goldberg were fervent advocates of the legalization of card playing among patients. Zealous administrators attempted to forbid the pastime because of the gambling that went along with it. Both men felt that "rules against card playing do not prevent secret gatherings. . . . The natural effects of prohibition are stealthy opposition and intensification of the desire."

A costume party at Purim was an old tradition at Montefiore. Goldberg was enthusiastic: "The fancy dress helps to release certain desires which otherwise would remain hidden. . . . There follows the belief in the prospect of a better state, and this indicates an advance on the road to recovery."

Outings to distant places were a feature of life at Montefiore for those in any condition to travel. Goldberg gave instructions: "In a city on a river, an annual boat ride will always be taken, accompanied by a doctor, nurse, and other assistants, for an all-day sail. Wheelchair patients can be transported to the landing on trucks, the others by taxi. At the landing, the steamer line will have to provide enough competent help to take the chairs down very carefully."

He made a special plea for the education of the children: "A hospital for chronic diseases should keep full step with all advances that have been effected in offsetting the possible retardation of developing childhood involved by an enforced stay in a hospital. This retardation is generally conceived as equivalent to so many pages torn out of the children's lives."

Dr. A. I. Ringer wrote about one of the patients who had spent many years at Montefiore, kept alive by good nursing care, a mystery to the physicians:

"Becky Kornreicher has been a patient at the Montefiore Hospital for a longer period than anyone can recall. Today, nobody looks up her early records. The pages of her early history have literally been worn to shreds from so much manipulation. Today, Becky is simply taken for granted. She is as much a part of the Montefiore Hospital as is the Zander Room or the Library.

"The best medical care had not stemmed the ravages of her disease. Her muscles withered, her bronze-colored skin clinging taut to her bones, her face mask-like and expressionless, her lips thin and drawn tight with a nose pinched almost to a point, she looked like an underdeveloped twelve-year-old girl, except for her eyes. These sparkled with native intelligence, sympathy, and kindness and disclosed the maturity of the woman.

"Becky had long ago lost the power of locomotion. Her arms and legs were merely stiff appendages. Her fingers were like wooden pencils sticking out of her hands. As she was put in her chair or bed, so she had to stay.

"Her mouth was fixed and partly open. When she talked, it sounded like a voice coming out of the loudspeaker of an old-fashioned radio. Her eyes, however, were the only part of her body that could move and talk. They were alive."

On the other hand, there were more and more patients for whom treatment was possible, including those with diabetes. A careful experimental program was a necessity. Not only were physicians ignorant of the long-term effects of insulin, but methods of manufacture were so uncertain that the strength of the hormone varied from batch to batch. There were so few legal restraints on human experimentation, and patients were so desperate for help, that there was no dearth of subjects. So many people received such immediate, dramatic help from insulin that acceptance was fast.

Diabetes is not a simple disease. Like tuberculosis, it affects many parts of the body, causing the degeneration of veins and, often, of eyesight. In many elderly people it is a mild, slow-moving condition, controllable by diet. Younger people suffer comas and ongoing damage to their bodies. In children, "juvenile onset diabetes," if untreated, is quickly fatal.

The manifold complications, the novelty of the treatment, and the continuing need for control of the diet required that sufferers remain in the hospital. One of those who remained the longest was A., who arrived at Montefiore in 1924 at the age of six. She stayed for ten years and then, for almost ten more years, was treated as an outpatient.

In 1923, A. had whooping cough and a few weeks later her mother noticed that she was drinking water and urinating frequently. Her appetite was poor and she began to lose weight. A friend advised her mother to have her urine tested for sugar, and a week later A. was admitted to Mount Sinai Hospital, where she suffered her first diabetic coma. After five months in Mount Sinai, A. came to Montefiore on February 1, 1924. The next day she was acutely ill with diarrhea, abdominal pains, and the typical acetone-smelling breath of the diabetic. She was given insulin and orange juice and in the early afternoon seemed better. At five o'clock she vomited, appearing much sicker and sleepier. In the first twenty-four hours she received 70 units of insulin.

A.'s diabetes was to prove always difficult to control. Three years later, her chart read: "It has been impossible to keep the patient on a satisfactory diet with insulin . . . and have patient free without hypoglycemic episodes."

Too young to understand the importance of diet, she was accused, in the doctor's notes, of "stealing food" or of "failure to consume all of weighed diet." A report of vomiting is followed by the note: "Was seen eating candy yesterday afternoon." Careful surveillance meant that she was often treated for conditions that in a normal child might have been allowed to run their course. On Christmas Eve 1925, her temperature shot up to 103 degrees. She was given an enema. Three days later, her temperature was down to normal and she was begging to get up. As would be expected after the enema, movements were not regular, so she was given daily purgatives "as well as enemas." On January 7, the doctor described her as "listless," a condition that might have been expected.

One night, when A. was twelve years old, the other children told an attendant that A. had a convulsion. The attendant found her lying prone with her arms and legs stretched out. She was breathing strangely. The attendant could not wake her and A. vomited a large amount of undigested spinach. By chance, a physician happened by and was told of the incident. He rushed in and found A. in a coma. He administered adrenalin, and A. sat up, vomited more spinach, and became "exceedingly irritable."

Doctors, nurses, and the social worker began to worry about the psychological damage being inflicted by this long hospital stay. Dr. Jack Masur decided that "in an attempt to rehabilitate her and to avoid protracted institutional life, we shall try a period of home care with Outpatient Department supervision weekly." A social worker visited her parents to make sure that they understood the diet needed. A. herself was taught how to measure and prepare her own food and how to give herself insulin injections. On December 4, 1934, fifteen-year-old A. went home.

The experiment was not entirely successful. For the next few years, A. lived partly at home and partly at Montefiore. The doctors' notes, however, referred, as they always had, to her "lack of cooperation" with her diet. By 1940, she was much sicker, entering Montefiore in May, not to leave until August. In September, she was readmitted for another month.

At twenty-one, the dark-eyed child had become an "obese young woman who looks and behaves younger than her stated age," who said that she had no interest in cooperating with the doctors. She had "ceased to care." In this mood of indifference she was admitted again because infections had developed at the site of the injections. The infection was successfully treated, but there was no cure for A.'s loss of hope. She died at Montefiore on November 21, 1942.

If A. had lived before the discovery of insulin she would have been dead within a few months of the first discovery of diabetes. Her purgatory of infections and comas and nausea and hunger provided the kind of information that helped thousands of others to live. During those same years, Montefiore was able to teach other patients to inject themselves, to control their own diets, and to live out satisfactory lives. Each year more and more patients were discharged to continue under the watchful eyes of the doctors in the Outpatient Clinics.

While Boas was running Montefiore, dealing with temperamental chiefs, attracting an enlarged and talented house staff, giving patients a voice in the running of the institution, raising a family, and attending to his own private practice, he was also tinkering with a useful invention, his cardiotachometer, a device for measuring the heartbeat over extended periods of time, under differing conditions.

The pulse rate and the heartbeat normally coincide, and both indicate the activity of the heart, in good and bad health. In the early seventeenth century Galileo made detailed measurements of the pulse rate, but not until after 1850 did doctors begin to count the beat of the patient's pulse as part of an ordinary physical examination. By the 1920s, the sphygmograph (which measures the pulse), the polygraph (the "lie detector," a device which measures a variety of physical responses including pulse rate and blood pressure), the electrocardiograph (which traces a graph showing the electric current produced by movements of the heart muscle), were all in general use. They had one common disadvantage. All were used when the patient was sitting quietly at rest. Boas wanted an instrument to measure the heartbeat of a patient moving around, performing various types of physical activity.

Devising a counter was not difficult. The problem lay in picking up the heartbeat. First, Boas and his friend Dr. Benjamin Liebowitz tried "an electrical contact, pneumatically actuated by the mechanical impulse of the heart or pulse beat." That didn't work because the slightest movement jarred the contact loose. They then tried a microphone, but any microphone sensitive enough to pick up the heartbeat also registered all kinds of extraneous noises.

Professor H. B. Williams of Columbia University suggested

that they try using the electrical current generated by the heart itself to power their counter. Dr. Alfred N. Goldsmith and other collaborators working with Boas found that having the patient put his or her fingers into jars of salty water was enough to establish the contact. The disadvantage again was that the patient had to remain perfectly still. They tried wet bandages wound around the arms and held in place by wire. That was effective until the bandages dried out. Finally, they settled on two small metal cups filled with green soap and sewn to elastic tapes which were tied around the chest, holding the cups in place over the heart.

Once that problem was solved, the inventors developed mechanisms for amplifying the sounds, recording them, and operating a counter which traced out the patterns for the heartbeat on a strip of paper that came out of the apparatus at the rate of 72 feet an hour.

Boas found that he could use wires up to 20 feet in length between the electrodes and the input jack of the amplifier, thus allowing the patient, or fellow experimenter, to move around with some freedom.

Patients and physicians at Montefiore were hooked up and their heartbeats recorded while "reading in bed," sleeping, "trying to sleep," eating, "half sitting in wheelchair," "sitting in wheelchair," running and doing calisthenics. Boas also measured the heartbeat of subjects during sex, thus providing fifty years of rumors as to the identity of the participants.

The original cardiotachometer is now in the Smithsonian Museum in recognition of the importance of this step in the progress of attempts to understand the workings of that pump upon which life depends.

Boas' relationships with influential people at Montefiore did not go as smoothly as his inventing. He had a habit of speaking the truth as he saw it. In his last annual report Boas spoke of a summer program for children with cardiac conditions. Charities, such as the Tribune Fresh Air Fund, which provided country vacations for city children refused to take children with heart problems. Mrs. Sol Stroock of the Ladies' Auxiliary was particularly interested in these children and she persuaded Mr. Marc H. Mack to donate $100,000 for the purchase of a farm-house as a vacation home for the children. Boas announced the gift but expressed doubts about the plan: "Whether this vacation work will lead further and actually have served to improve the resistance of these children to the point that they will better resist the progress of their heart disease is doubtful judging from the experience of other cardiac convalescent homes."

Boas was never willing to confuse social welfare and actual medicine, in spite of his realization of the need for both, and he was never ready to flatter his audience by modifying his honest point of view. (His successor never expressed anything but absolute enthusiasm for Big Tree Farm.)

The Board of Trustees had learned to look somewhat askance at their young Director, so blunt and so busy with so many projects. By the beginning of 1928, it was obvious that Boas' view of his appropriate role at Montefiore differed from that of the Board. In February, he wrote to S. G. Rosenbaum: "I have given further thought to the matter which we have had under discussion, and have regretfully come to the conclusion that, in view of the fact that the Board does not favor giving me further opportunities for my medical development, it will be wisest for me to resign." The Board of Trustees accepted his resignation, asking him to stay on for a period of six to nine months.

At the annual meeting in 1928, Rosenbaum announced the completion of the new sanitarium along with plans for further construction: expansion of the Schiff Pavilion for custodial cases, a new building exclusively for children, and a new research building. These dreams, alas, were all to fall victim to the Great Depression. Other changes announced at the same meeting were to have a longer life: three women were to be added to that all-male Board: Mrs. Dore Felbel, Mrs. Robert Isaac, and Mrs. Sol M. Stroock.

Rosenbaum also announced the appointment of a new Director.

CHAPTER
11
Ephraim Michael Bluestone

As successor to Boas, the Trustees looked for a man (no woman was ever considered) who would devote his full-time effort to administration, not distracted by his own patients or by an enthusiasm for research. Maurice Fishberg found him. With his assimilationist views, Fishberg was no Zionist, but, alarmed by the signs of the cardiac problems that were to kill him at the age of sixty-four, he decided that he wanted to visit the land of his fathers before he died. In Palestine, he met a young physician, Ephraim Michael Bluestone, who was spending a turbulent two years as director of the Hadassah Medical Organization, then attempting to serve the young settlements.

Bluestone was temperamentally unfitted to the chaotic atmosphere of sectarian argument and physical violence that was Palestine at the time. An agnostic in religion, he was disapproving of the observances of Orthodoxy; a political moderate, he was uninterested in the feverish discussions of socialist theory; socially reserved, he disliked the communal intimacy of the kibbutzim. Always rigid in his opinions, he could not brook opposition. Bluestone, trained in the stately atmosphere of New York's Mount Sinai, was unprepared for the rowdy lines of union pickets outside his office in the sunshine of the promised land.

Finding much in common with Fishberg, Bluestone responded positively to the invitation to come to the Bronx as the new Director. At Montefiore he followed the tradition of Baruch and Boas in his deep concern for social issues. Emotionally he was very different from either. A group of hospital administrators introduced themselves to each other at a conference, exchanging first names. A stranger asked, "And what do they call you, Dr. Bluestone?" The answer came, cold and firm: "Dr. Bluestone."

They did. Everybody who worked with or for Ephraim Michael Bluestone treated him with respectful formality at all times. Dignified and distant in manner, he was handsome in the carefully manicured movie-star look of the thirties, with sleek hair, styled moustache, pin-striped suit, conservative tie, always carefully posed in photographs. His attitudes toward personal behavior at times recalled those of the previous century. The divorce of a friend or acquaintance was always spoken of as a somewhat shocking occurrence. Fifty years later, he still remembered with disapproval the drink with which Boas welcomed him to Montefiore "even though Prohibition was the law."

His penny pinching became a legend. A newly hired division chief made the mistake of writing a quick note to the Director on the nearest white space at hand, a file card, and received in reply a sharp memo pointing out the high cost of such material. He was calm, aloof, careful, and in the habit of looking out of his office window onto Gun Hill Road, watching for late-arriving employees. His thrifty handling of money steered Montefiore through the financial shoals of the thirties. He was married, but had no children, and sometimes found it hard to understand the pressing financial needs of the young doctors who rejected his advice that they should save half their stipends.

And yet, beneath his prim exterior beat the heart of a revolutionary. A man opposed for sixty years to the concept of medicine as a marketplace commodity, he spent his professional life devising new methods for the delivery of health care that aimed at changing the economic structure of that delivery. His one year of private practice "scared and scarred" him. From then on, he was determined to find other ways of paying doctors, and other ways of enabling patients to afford necessary medical attention. Toward the end of his life, he said in an interview: "I am an opponent of the fee-for-service principle. It leads to all kinds of dreadful things: splitting fees, unnecessary surgery. It affects the hospital structure because the man who calls in consultants is favored." The poor were always with him. At Montefiore, the patients, if not originally poor, had been brought to that state by the insatiable demands of chronic illness. Sharing George Bernard Shaw's belief that the basic flaw in medical practice is economic, he created programs whose purpose was to correct that error.

Bluestone always saw any hospital as a forbidding, frightening, dangerous place.

He was equally wary of the fee-for-service medicine that dominated the American scene and was so staunchly defended by the American Medical Association. His one year of private practice showed him the suffering imposed on poor families by the economics of medicine in the days when there was no widespread system of health-care insurance. The experience also convinced him that his interest lay in administration, not in the personal, direct tendering of care, and he never again practiced as a physician.

The Board of Trustees was happy that he would not be distracted from his administrative role. They wanted a full-time Director. And so E. M. Bluestone became the first non-practicing physician to be Director of Montefiore.

Bluestone obtained his M.D. from the College of Physicians and Surgeons in 1916. He served as a first lieutenant in the Laboratory Service of the Medical Corps of the United States Army in France. After the overseas adventure came that one unhappy year of private practice from which he was rescued by a chance meeting on the subway with a friend who told him of an opening in administration in Mount Sinai Hospital. There he became assistant director to the man he admired all his life, S. S. Goldwater. For six years he sat at the feet of the hospital administrator who, he felt, invented the discipline. In 1926, he went to Palestine as director of the Hadassah Medical Organization.

The institution on Gun Hill Road to which Bluestone was summoned occupied sixteen acres of lawns and flower-filled gardens and handsome brick buildings, surrounded by farms and the beginnings of residential development, on the far northern borders of New York City. The buildings were now fifteen years old, and Bluestone vigorously set about modernizing the institution. In ten years—in the depths of the Great Depression —he spent $350,000 improving the physical plant and incidentally making space for eighty-five more beds. He took advantage of New York City's make-work projects for some additions such as a bandstand on the lawn for outdoor concerts. He upgraded the administrative and housekeeping staff, rigorously rooting out corruption.

The first Chairman of the Board under whom Bluestone served was Fred Stein. A reserved, austere man, his attitudes in personal matters resembled Bluestone's. More importantly, he and Bluestone shared a vision of the hospital and an appreciation of the role of all those other services which sustained a reasonable life for the sick. In 1933, Bluestone wrote to Stein: "Dr. Nemet called this afternoon to talk over a rather urgent medical problem that I have been discussing with you and Mr. Moses off and on for almost five years. It relates to the case of patients discharged from the cardio-vascular service of the medical division. At the present time patients are discharged from the medical wards and, if they are not cared for in our follow-up clinic, or if they are not favored with a home visit by one of the doctors under the special fund recently made available by the Ladies' Auxiliary Society, they are apt to return to us with a relapse in a comparatively short time." Bluestone wanted to use Big Tree Farm as a convalescent home to provide for further care. But during the Depression, the money was not available.

Henry Moses, who became the Chairman of the Board in 1936, was quite different. A man who had devoted his life to making money, he approached the medical world with the same tough and aggressive need to understand its structure as he had used in his approach to banking and finance, sharing Bluestone's desire for expansion and for finding outstanding chiefs of services.

Before he became Chairman, he was Chairman of the Medical Committee. In both positions, he was fond of giving dinners for the staff at which he solicited their opinions on hospital matters. On March 14, 1931, he gave a dinner for the Medical Board. The discussion dealt with almost every problem and point of view affecting the medical staff. Amalgamation of Montefiore with other Jewish hospitals (Bronx and Lebanon) and nursing homes in the Bronx was floated as an idea—one of the great recurring themes of attempts to rationalize and regionalize health care in the borough.

Israel Wechsler was more concerned about education, talking about the hope of a Jewish medical school while doubting that the "tremendous financial support necessary" would ever be available. He pointed out "the inefficiency, the sham, and the tawdriness" of graduate study in New York. Only in neurology had the connection with Columbia provided for "adequate training" at Montefiore.

The path followed by neurology at Montefiore was indicated by Wechsler's proposal that "a fellowship in neurophysiology be provided to enable the study of neurology along the latest approved lines of study, that is, physiological, physical-chemical and bio-chemical." Dr. Harold Neuhof, on the other hand, was suspicious of an emphasis on teaching, stating firmly that "it is the duty of the attending staff to concentrate their attention on the patients. Their time should not be devoted to teaching under the present organization, for it tends to leave too much of the responsibility of the care of patients to members of the resident staff." Dr. A. A. Schwartz, disagreeing, "informed the group that

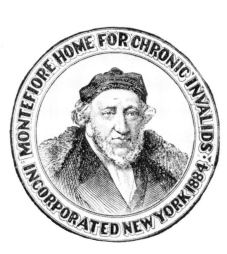

Jewish communities all over the world erected charitable institutions to honor the one hundredth birthday of Sir Moses Montefiore. The Home had its own seal with his likeness

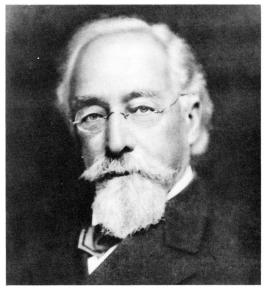

Simon Baruch, M.D., the first Chairman of the Medical Board, fought for active medical care for all patients

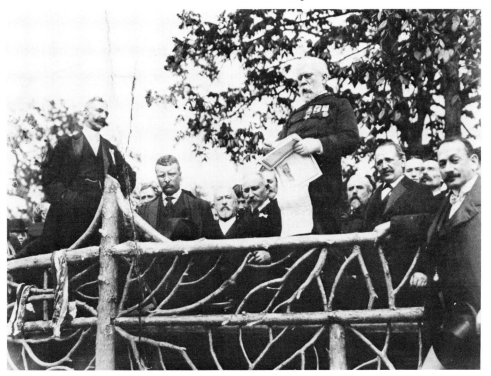

Teddy Roosevelt, then Vice-President of the United States, attended the opening of Montefiore's Country Sanitarium. Seated next to him was Jacob Schiff, investment banker and the most powerful Jewish leader in the country. As President of the Board of Trustees for thirty-five years, he emphasized both science and social concern as the twin cornerstones of Montefiore

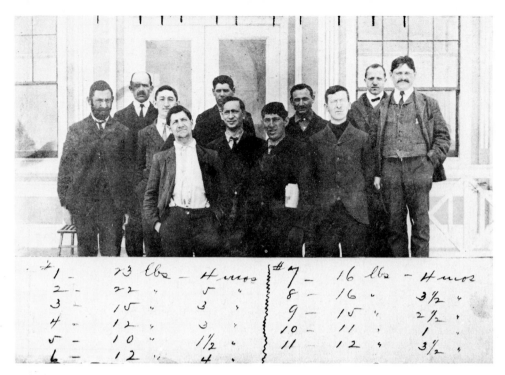

#1 -	23 lbs -	4 mos		#7 -	16 lbs -	4 mos
2 -	22 "	5 "		8 -	16 "	3½ "
3 -	15 "	3 "		9 -	15 "	2½ "
4 -	12 "	3 "		10 -	11 "	1 "
5 -	10 "	1½ "		11 -	12 "	3½ "
6 -	12 "	4 "				

Careful records were kept of the weight gained by each patient at the Country Sanitarium, since a loss of weight was one of the symptoms of tuberculosis, and the opposite a sign of recovery

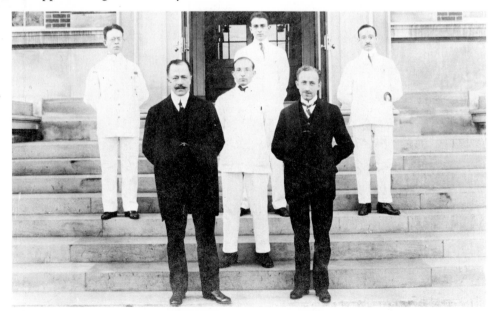

Administration and House Staff, 1915

Siegfried Wachsmann, M.D., Medical Director, with frock coat and curled mustaches, stands on the front steps with his assistant, M. W. Goldstein, M.D., and the four residents who cared for 650 patients

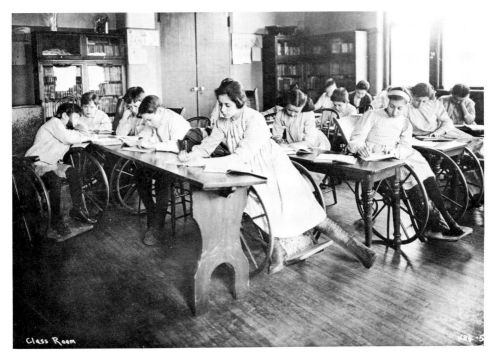

The children's classroom in the Montefiore Hospital for Chronic Diseases was part of the New York City public school system

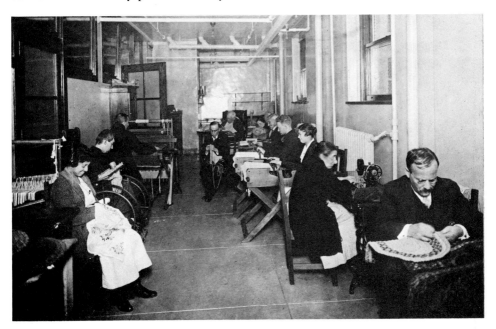

The Occupational Therapy Workroom in 1919. The man in front making a rag mat suffered from meningomyelitis. The Director of Occupational Therapy reported that he was "greatly depressed and very indifferent on first coming to the workroom. Now habitually cheerful and takes great interest in keeping the workmanship up to a high standard"

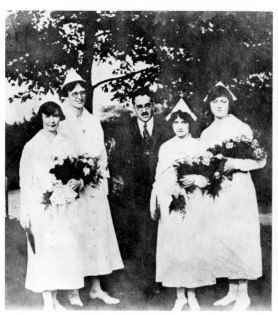

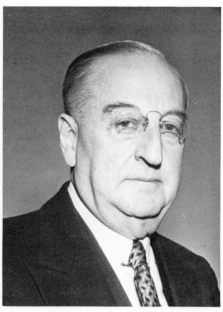

Ernst Boas, M.D., Medical Director of the Montefiore Hospital for Chronic Diseases, 1920–28, with Mildred Constantine, Director of the School of Nursing, and the first graduates of the school, Anne C. Donahue, Bertha V. Bokser, and Irma Y. Reiser

Henry Moses, President of the Board of Trustees, collaborated with Bluestone as Director in bringing about the changes which set Montefiore on the path to becoming a general hospital dealing with every kind of illness

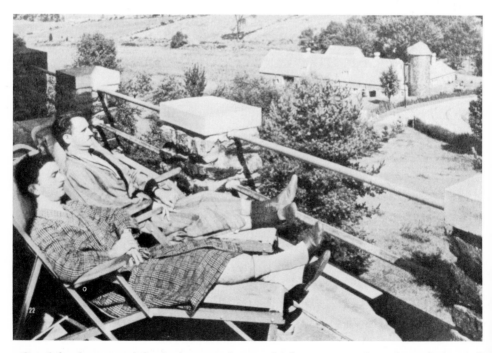

Good food, rest, and fresh air were the standard treatments for tuberculosis until after World War II and the advent of antibiotics

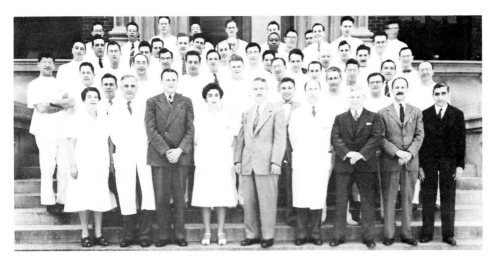

Administrators and House Staff, 1947

Front row: Ruth Lubliner, M.D., later Pathologist to Morrisania Hospital; Daniel Laszlo, Chief of the Cancer Division; Henry Makover, M.D.; Naomi De Sola Pool, M.D.; E. M. Bluestone, M.D., Director of Montefiore 1928–50; Louis Leiter, M.D., Chief of Medicine; Harry Zimmerman, M.D., Chief of Pathology; Samuel Rosen, M.D., a pathologist who worked with David Marine; and Emil Bauman, Marine's chief chemist.

The early postwar years brought a flood of talented residents to Montefiore and this house staff includes such people as Isador Rossman, M.D.; Harold Rifkin, M.D.; and Julius Parker, M.D., all of whom played an important role in the building of the modern Montefiore. Bluestone began bringing black residents to his hospital in the early thirties, when they were not being accepted at most hospitals in the United States.

By 1982, house staff throughout the Medical Center numbered 622, impossible to include in a single photograph

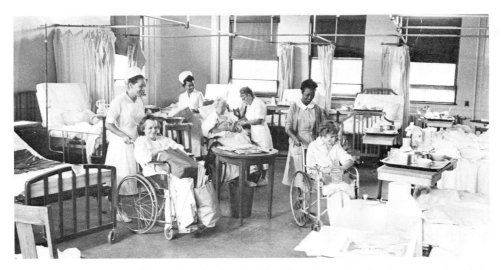

Until the late 1950s, Montefiore's chronically ill patients lived in long wards with thirty or forty beds each

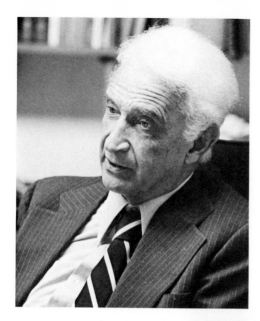

Martin Cherkasky, M.D., who led Montefiore from 1951 to 1981, during the institution's greatest period of growth and development

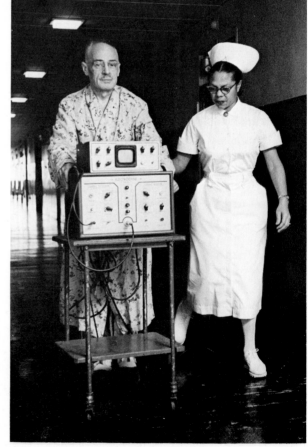

Pincus Shapiro, a seventy-six-year-old retired salesman, was the first patient to leave a hospital after treatment with a transvenous pacemaker. A fifty-foot extension cord allowed him to take short walks, pushing his pacemaker ahead of him

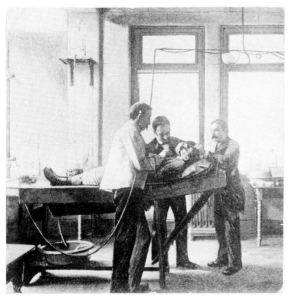

While surgeons talked of "antiseptic techniques," this view of the operating room in 1889 suggests that they were not always observed

The modern operating room scarcely has room for all the machines and all the people required for intricate surgery

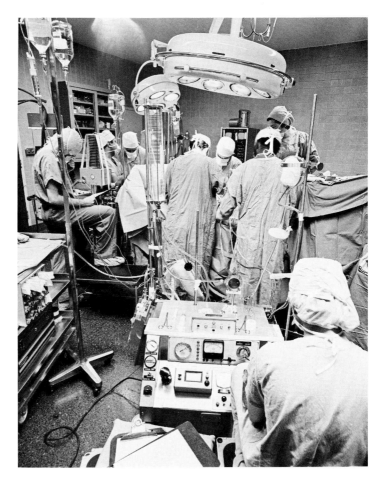

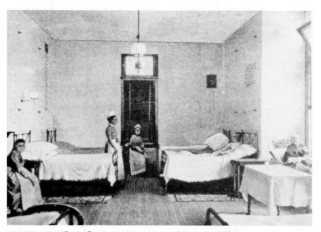

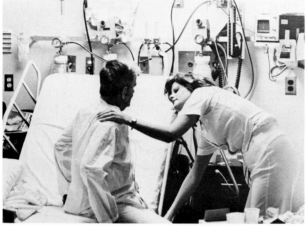

The wards in 1889 were bare. Modern nursing care
depends on human concern, technology, and a high
level of education

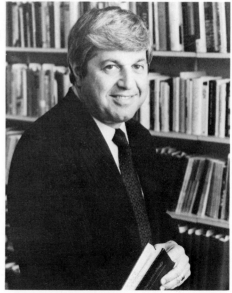

Carl Eisdorfer, Ph.D., M.D., the psychiatrist who became President of
Montefiore Medical Center in 1981

the wealth of clinical material at Montefiore Hospital is largely wasted and that the demonstration of this material during the course of rounds would in no way take away from the care of the patients."

One of the most interesting statements of the evening was made by Dr. H. T. Hyman, who "pointed out the failure of the present medical organization to consider the patient as a social, medical and economic problem," and cited many instances of neglect in dealing with the patients from these points of view.

Summing up and commenting on the evening, Bluestone stated that "no matter what form the expansion would take, the result would be a Montefiore Hospital which would admit all types of patients, including the acute, the chronic and the aged, limiting their stay in accordance with their need for hospital service and following them up as often as necessary thereafter." Economics and war were to delay the dream. The disaster of the Great Depression weighed heavily on Bluestone and his hospital in a country without a safety net of social services, welfare payments, unemployment insurance, food stamps, or any mechanism for paying for medical care for the poor.

Bluestone coped with tight Depression budgets by urging all his administrators and division chiefs to cut expenses wherever possible, and he slashed salaries of the housekeeping and clerical help, people who traditionally earned less than their equivalents in industry. During the thirties, they were to suffer from a series of reductions in already meager paychecks.

In 1932, the School of Nursing was closed, the official announcement reflecting the various elements that had gone into the decision. In the first place, the school was declared to be an "expensive . . . educational experiment," the exchange of service in return for training felt to be unequal, since, apart from the four months spent as a preliminary student, the nurse in training spent, in actuality, only one full year at Montefiore, the rest of her time being taken up with acute-care experience at Bellevue and Long Island College Hospitals and with vacations. Secondly, the combination of the post-World War I overproduction of nurses and the Depression had produced enormous unemployment among graduate nurses. There were now over 2,200 training schools in the United States, turning out, in 1931, 30,000 graduates at a time when there were 25,000 nurses looking for jobs in the New York area alone.

Bluestone understood, however, the fundamental dilemma faced by the nursing profession in the thirties, the fact that most graduate nurses would never find steady jobs, or any jobs at all, as long as hospitals were staffed by cheap student labor. He promised that at Montefiore "full-time nurses will be employed to take the place of the students-in-training." He hoped that many other nursing schools would close.

With less money coming from philanthropy, the new technologies for treating patients placed additional burdens on tight budgets. In 1929, Montefiore acquired its first oxygen tent. Soon hospital administrators were complaining about the high cost of novel procedures in the same way that forty years earlier they had anguished over the price of rubber gloves or fifty years later were to suffer over million-dollar CAT scanners. Bluestone was especially troubled over the cost of blood transfusions, which were increasing in number in light of the growing understanding of surgical shock and the need to replace blood.

The dilemma affected Bluestone only when the patient could not afford to pay: "Where the patient can finance his own treatment the question does not reach the administrator." His own attitude was that "the community must provide for the poor patient," and he never lost his awareness that, as long as low-income patients were dependent upon charity for their care, they were in danger of being exploited by hospitals, used indiscriminately as "teaching material." Many of Bluestone's little homilies addressed to fellow administrators were intended to protect patients and to warn against the machinations of doctors.

Bluestone mistrusted physicians; he was also fully aware that medical care was only one component in the formula that kept patients alive. These two ideas resulted in the unusual degree of respect that he accorded the other professionals within the Hospital. He always spoke admiringly of Lenna Cooper, the dietician he brought in from Battle Creek. About Minnie Smith, "headworker" of the Social Service Department when he arrived at Montefiore, Bluestone remarked: "So far as I know, she never had any formal schooling in her profession, perhaps because this was not the fashion at the time. She had learned from daily exposure, in a voluntary general hospital which was unique in the history of medicine as being solely devoted to the continued scientific care of patients suffering from prolonged illness— curable and incurable—under a demanding related program of social service."

Bluestone welcomed the new college-trained generation of social workers to Montefiore, and they found him supportive of them as professionals. Bess Dana, who was to become a professor in community medicine at Mount Sinai, came to Montefiore in the forties and found: "In most hospitals at that time the social workers walked two paces behind the doctors. Not at Montefiore. Bluestone thought we were important."

Bluestone asserted: "It is literally impossible for the modern physician to practice his profession without help in one form or another from the social worker." This was no mere suggestion that the social worker should join the nurse as "handmaiden" to the physician. Bluestone was talking about a quite different approach to patient care, the opposite of the physician-dominated mode that was the norm in American hospitals. He wanted a hospital where "the doctor is the medical technician working in an atmosphere of social service, thinking beyond his prescription of medicine or the surgical operation. The major portion of any 'cure' is a social matter which has broader and more fundamental implications than the actual medical and surgical treatment of a case."

His own experience left Bluestone with a continuing concern for the struggles of young doctors at a time when interns and residents received no salary at all and were frequently forced by economic pressures into dubious decisions at the beginning of a professional career. During his first year at Montefiore, he was visited by the cousin of a surgeon he had known in Palestine. The visitor announced that he wanted to make a contribution to the hospital, beginning with $1,200. Bluestone said: "I thought the best use for the contribution was to give the interns some pin money so that they would not be so dependent on their parents." The Board of Trustees agreed. The idea was well received, and when the donated money ran out, the Board added enough to the budget to pay interns $25 a month and residents $50.

For young doctors, the problems of making a living did not end on graduation from house staff status, and Bluestone's concern continued. Some were paid "Fellowship Stipends" of $50, $100, or $200 a month and put to work in the research labs. Others were sent overseas to study. Bluestone found help for other fledglings in the form of part-time salaried jobs in nursing homes and other institutions.

Bluestone found a solution for one of the problems that had plagued Boas. The physical isolation of Montefiore in the twenties and thirties made for difficulties in providing the best possible care for patients. Most of the doctors officially listed as staff members were also on the staff of Mount Sinai. Their private practices were in Manhattan. The time they gave to Montefiore was voluntary, and with the long distance to be traveled by subway or the uncertain and expensive automobile, many spent very little time on Gun Hill Road. This accident of geography was helpful to Bluestone in persuading the Board of Trustees to embark on the great experiment of the full-time principle in medicine.

In 1913, Johns Hopkins had made full-time appointments in medicine, pediatrics, and surgery. Other medical schools slowly followed but, in hospitals, full-time appointments were rare when on August 19, 1929, the Board of Trustees of Montefiore resolved that the "position of Chief of the Medical Division be established on a full-time basis." B. S. Oppenheimer was the incumbent, and his retirement three years later provided Bluestone with the chance to implement both the full-time principle and another of his plans for Montefiore, that of attracting full-time chiefs and other staff of international reputation.

The rise of the Nazis in Europe, forcing many great physicians into exile, assisted him in this latter dream. Bluestone's first choice for a new Chief of Medicine was Dr. Isidore Snapper of the University of Amsterdam. Dr. Snapper, however, suggested that Dr. Leopold Lichtwitz of the University of Berlin be approached in his stead. Dr. Lichtwitz readily accepted the position.

Leopold Lichtwitz had been director of the Medical Service at the Rudolf Virchow Hospital in Berlin. At Montefiore, although the appointment as Chief of Medicine was theoretically part-time, he served almost full-time, becoming deeply involved in research as well as patient care. Dr. Michael Ringer admired Lichtwitz and his impact: "He was a top-flight clinician and a great teacher. He attracted a better-trained and more ambitious attending staff and interns. A friendly, although respectful relationship between chief and staff emerged, so that his influence augmented the gains toward the development of a full-time teaching hospital."

The fact that Montefiore's patients rarely provided any income to physicians also aided the process of putting doctors on salary, and enabled Bluestone to strike a decisive blow against fee-for-service medicine. In that era, full-time salaried practice made particularly good sense in Jewish hospitals. Few Jewish doctors could hope for prestigious academic appointments at medical schools. Full-time salaried hospital positions provided time for teaching, facilities for research, and a supply of students. The other Jewish hospitals in New York gradually followed Bluestone's lead, with the Federation of Jewish Philanthropies willing to provide the money. Refugees from American medical schools joined the refugees from Hitler's Europe to provide a remarkable concentration of intelligence and excellence in the Federation hospitals.

Bluestone continued the Montefiore tradition of accepting women into the house staff and went one step further. He took on the first black residents. One year during the thirties, he actually had a black woman on the house staff—at a time when either of those attributes was an automatic disqualification in most American hospitals.

Almost half of Montefiore's patients in the Bronx and Bedford suffered from tuberculosis. Fishberg died in 1934, and four years later, Max Pinner was appointed full-time Chief of the Division of Pulmonary Diseases, firmly establishing the full-time principle as a basic part of the structure of medical care at Montefiore.

Pinner graduated from the University of Tübingen in 1919, and after two years' work in Hamburg came to the United States, where he served as the director of the laboratory in the Municipal Tuberculosis Sanitarium of Chicago and then in a similar position in Detroit. From there he went to Arizona as associate director in charge of laboratories and research in the Desert Sanitarium of Tucson and then back East as principal pathologist in the New York State District Tuberculosis Hospitals.

With Marine, the full-time chief he inherited, Bluestone carried on a never-ending discussion about the relative responsibilities of the various laboratories within the Hospital and the sometimes conflicting demands of patient care and research. Bluestone was never quite sure how to handle his resident genius. In general, however, their attitudes toward money were similar. Both were capable of monumental thriftiness, Marine always careful to return whatever amount of a grant remained unspent at the end of an experiment.

While he sometimes appeared austere and aloof, Marine loved to teach and enjoyed students. Dr. Dennison Young remembers: "You had to make up your mind that if you went to see him, you wouldn't get any work done because he loved to talk . . . but he was very sweet, very kind, very interested in the younger men coming up."

He was generous with recognition of the work of those who labored with him, his annual reports full of listings of, and tributes to, their publications. Over the years, many women worked in his labs as physicians and technicians. In 1931, of twenty "employees" in the lab, twelve were women. When reporting on the year's activities he was always careful to indicate the sex of the investigator.

In an environment where the primacy of the M.D. is often jealously guarded, Marine treasured all qualifications. The chemist Emil J. Baumann, Ph.D., who came to Montefiore with Marine and outlasted him there, was reputed to know more about the chemistry of iodine than any other living being. He took over during Marine's occasional absences and sometimes appeared an even more forbidding presence, a man who went on wearing celluloid collars for many years after they had been abandoned by the rest of the world.

Another vital member of the team was Harry Hawker, whose skilled hands produced many of the tools used in the labs. Instruments for research had not yet become big business. Harry Hawker, trained in England as a jeweler, became Marine's general factotum, handyman, and mechanic. His experience with jewelry gave him an ideal background for precision work, and he flourished as toolmaker, carpenter, glass blower, tinsmith, plumber, steamfitter, and anything else required.

In 1930, the New York Academy of Medicine struck a gold medal to be awarded annually to "the outstanding man of science in the medical profession in America." The first year the recipient was Freud's friend Carl Koller, still a consulting ophthalmologist at Montefiore, in recognition of his discoveries in the use of cocaine as a local anesthetic. The next year, David Marine was honored. Marine made four great contributions to medicine and science. Three of these—the establishment of iodine as necessary for thyroid function (1907), the proposal of iodine as therapy for Grave's disease (1911), and the introduction of iodine prophylaxis (1917)—were the result of work done before he came to Montefiore. The fourth, the description of cyanide goiter, came out of the laboratories at Montefiore.

When lists are made of scientists whose work should have been rewarded with a Nobel Prize but was not, Marine's name is frequently mentioned, and not just because of his dazzling discovery. The years of careful, detailed, painstaking exploration that followed were as valuable. At Montefiore he left a tradition of a Division of Laboratories dedicated to research and education in a particular field, a field large enough to offer insight into the fundamentals of human existence. And he left a tradition of a division working in close collaboration with other specialties in exploring new modalities of patient care.

Under Bluestone there was a rapid expansion of the outpatient clinics. Most of the clinics remained providers of follow-up care, designed to help former patients, not to bring in new patients. The staffing also reflected Bluestone's interest in using other professions. Each clinic had the services of a social worker. A pattern developed of patients spending time in the hospital, being released and cared for as outpatients, returning to hospital beds when they needed acute care, and being released again when the episode was over and the illness under control again. Former patients always had first preference for beds. Thus, the staff was gaining in experience in caring for patients over long periods of time in a variety of settings—as both inpatients and outpatients—the modern pattern for the care of chronic illness.

The coming of insulin released many diabetics from hospital beds to an active life while at the same time they required continuing medical supervision. (In these early years of the new treatment, the idea of patients giving themselves hypodermic injections was so radical that many came back to the hospital each day for their shots.) In the early thirties, some cardiac patients benefited in the same way from the first new effective drugs for the heart and circulation since the discovery of digitalis in the eighteenth century.

In many cardiac conditions, one of the most troubling and dangerous side effects is edema, the swelling caused by the collection of fluid in various parts of the body. If the left side of the heart is affected, fluid is likely to lodge in the lungs; problems on the right side lead to a gradual swelling of the whole body, beginning at the ankles. The burden of fluid adds to the difficulties of the heart in pumping blood through the body and can in itself prove fatal. A great leap forward in the treatment of heart patients was the introduction of diuretics, drugs which stepped up the production of urine and drained off the fluid. The first diuretic used on a large scale at Montefiore was urea, a salt prepared from urine. The dosage required was large, often about 18 grams a day dissolved in water, and urea has a most unpleasant taste. In spite of this, Drs. H. R. Miller and A. Feldman reported that most Montefiore patients "took the drug without remonstrance." Other patients, less desperate or less amenable to discipline, required coaxing.

The loss of fluid in patients was spectacular. One young woman was admitted to Montefiore six times between 1923 and 1927 suffering from chronic rheumatic cardiovascular disease. In 1929, she again entered the hospital at the age of twenty-eight. On digitalis alone she grew steadily worse. When urea, up to 56 grams a day, was added, her weight dropped from 135 to 114. Other patients had equally spectacular weight losses. The treatment was soon to be made obsolete by newer and more effective diuretics. The value of the experiments at Montefiore lay in the possibility of studying the effect of diuretics over long intervals of time. For instance, J.R. came to Montefiore on March 12, 1927, during one of a series of recurrent attacks of congestive heart failure. For the first twenty-nine days no urea was given, only digitalis. Then he took urea for 108 days. For 152 days urea was withheld, but then was given again for 732 days.

Soon, similar studies were being done on the newer diuretics, which were mercurial compounds. There had been suggestions from other researchers that these remedies were dangerous. Leonard Tarr and Sheldon Jacobson studied the effects of more than 3,000 injections of Salyrgan at Montefiore and were able to report that only five patients experienced ill effects, none of them serious. Of the thirty cases that came to autopsy, only one showed a lesion that might have been the result of mercury poisoning. Careful studies like these gave other physicians a firm base on which to proceed with their use of diuretics.

Many of the cardiac patients had a history of frequent re-admission to the Hospital. Dr. Meyer Friedenson attempted to use the lessons that were learned on the wards to keep these patients out of the Hospital: "The aim of our follow-up clinic has been to enable the patient to lead a comfortable existence at home and to relieve the mental attitude of the hopeless invalid by delaying his readmission to the hospital as long as is possible without sacrificing his best interests." He also used the argument that Dr. Bluestone was later to use in justifying his Home Care Program: "As a fair percentage of these individuals can be successfully treated as outpatients, and their inevitable readmission to the hospital be postponed, a considerable number of beds became available for others who need them."

Making sure that patients remembered to take their medication and stick to their diets was difficult. The dosage of digitalis that was effective varied from patient to patient and from day to day. Dr. Friedenson enlisted the patient in regulating the amount: "The patient is instructed to watch for nausea or vomiting, when he is to omit digitalis for one day, and then commence with a smaller daily dose. . . . Many patients in this way learn to gauge exactly the required dose by steering between nausea and vomiting on one hand, and dyspnea and palpitation on the other." Dr. Friedenson was enthusiastic about diuretics but believed that low-salt diet and the restriction of fluids was also necessary. Here again, education of the patient was the first requirement: "It is not sufficient to tell a patient, 'Don't drink much water,' and 'Cut out salt.' The patient requires specific directions."

There were more clinics involved with following up tuberculosis patients. The popularity in the thirties of pneumothorax treatments required an expansion of the facilities. Air was pumped into the chest cavity to prevent one lung from expanding, in the belief that this lung would thus be allowed to rest and, therefore, heal. After release from the Hospital the patient had to return to the clinic for periodic "refills," as Bluestone described the process, by the pneumothorax machine. In 1934, fifteen or twenty patients attended the Wednesday clinic and were taken care of by one machine. By 1937, there were so many patients that an additional clinic was held on Saturday mornings and three machines added. There were also special clinics for routine follow-up of tuberculosis, for chest taps, for gastric examination of T.B. patients, and for those who had both tuberculosis and diabetes, and the salvarsan clinic for patients with syphilis continued.

Clinics were set up to deal not only with the patients' major illnesses but with the secondary complaints that complicated their lives. An orthopedic clinic was established in 1934, allergy in 1935, and podiatry in 1936. There were also ear, nose, and throat, gynecological, genitourinary, gastrointestinal, skin, and radiotherapy clinics.

CHAPTER

12

Politics, Patients, and War

Less than ten years after Bluestone came to Montefiore, the man who was ultimately to succeed him arrived for his first sojourn as a resident. With smooth green lawns and flower-filled gardens, white cloths on the tables in the doctors' dining room, the pace of medicine as placid as the landscaping, the average patient stayed six months. Martin Cherkasky described the atmosphere of the institution when he arrived there in 1937: "It was leisurely. It was classical medicine. When you read the textbooks they show 'classical matters.' If you have rheumatic heart disease and disease of the valves of the heart as a result of rheumatic fever, in the textbooks it will show you the classical disease in full flower. You don't see that in the practice of medicine. As a young doctor, you try to hear the sounds that you're supposed to hear when you have a mitral stenosis. The mitral valve has been calcified; it doesn't function properly. You're supposed to hear a presystolic murmur. Well, you don't know whether you're hearing it or you're imagining it, because you see patients at an earlier clinical stage. You have to have an awful lot of experience and have heard a lot to understand what that's all about. That wasn't the case at Montefiore. When you came to Montefiore Hospital, you saw disease so advanced that it was unbelievable. We used to say that you could hear the presystolic murmur without putting your stethoscope in your ears."

Prolonged bed rest was an important and accepted therapy for many conditions, including most cardiac difficulties. Effective drug treatments were few. Cancer was treated with surgery, X-rays, and radium. Nevertheless, this was relatively inexpensive medicine. The 1,728 patients admitted cost $85,140.88 each year in "medical expenses," less than $50 each. The total daily cost for each patient was $4.14. Less than 15 percent of the days of care were paid for by patients at a time when 70 percent of the income of most voluntary hospitals came from fees.

Assigned to the Medical Division, Cherkasky joined the other thirty-four members of the house staff, divided into interns, assistant residents, and residents of the Medical, Surgical, Neurological, and Tuberculosis Divisions, Neuropathology, Pathology, Radiotherapy, Dermatology, Roentgenology, the Dental Service, and the Private Pavilion.

House officers were assigned to double rooms. Women lived in the Nurses' Residence, and "man" remained the normal synonym for resident or intern. A handbook rule stated: "Each man is off duty every other night and every Sunday."

"Members of the house staff are expected to act like ladies and gentlemen at all times, both on and off duty. There are no other rules in this Hospital governing conduct."

The rules came from the "Precedent Book," which at intervals the Hospital published and distributed to staff, a wonderful mishmash of information and instruction on such diverse subjects as vacations, special diets, preparing a body for the morgue, the use of the tennis courts, the metric system, the admission and discharge of patients, the contents of surgical carts, the duties of pantrymen—and innumerable other aspects of hospital life and work.

Bluestone added his own gloss to some rules. Boas, under "Duties of Nurse in Charge of Ward," included: "Be responsible for the ventilation of the ward." The new Director added to that: "Bad odors mean bad nursing."

Martin Cherkasky had attended medical school in Philadelphia during the Depression. The misery of the country was obvious to him. At Montefiore, he found other people deeply affected by the state of the country: "This was the first time that I'd ever come into a highly politicized atmosphere. I found here a group of very sophisticated, very well-organized political activists; in 1937 and 1938 we were right in the midst of the Spanish Civil War. It was a time of political and social movement. It was a desperate period because of economic problems, 25–30 percent unemployment, poverty, but clearly that was a period of great social gains. It was one of the great bursts in the history of this country, and I found a home at Montefiore. I used to quip that house officers at Montefiore were divided into two groups: half of them were at the hospital and half of them were at Madison Square Garden for the rallies."

The Chief of Medicine was not a figure who would necessarily appeal to the younger residents. In many ways, Lichtwitz was a figure from the past. In 1819, René Théophile Hyacinthe Laënnec published his account of the piece of medical technology he had invented—the stethoscope. Laënnec's instrument was a straight wooden cylinder. By the nineties the stethoscope had assumed its modern form. In the 1930s Lichtwitz walked the wards of Montefiore with a simple wooden cylinder—with one earpiece—that Laënnec would have recognized. He was doubly suspicious of newer inventions. Cherkasky was treating a young woman with Hodgkin's disease. Sulfanilamide was now available at Montefiore, and Cherkasky wanted to use it on his patient to battle a secondary infection. Lichtwitz would not agree. He forbade the experiment, maintaining that these new drugs were "a passing fad." The patient continued to suffer, and Cherkasky remembered Lichtwitz forever as "the only man who ever made me cry."

After finishing his year of residency, Cherkasky went on a trip to Europe with two other house officers. They traveled from London to Leningrad by ship, through the tension-ridden Kiel

Canal. They saw Odessa, Kiev, Tiflis, and Yalta; they were in Paris as the Munich settlement was announced, watching Europe slipping into the inferno. Cherkasky was not to return to Montefiore until the fires were extinguished.

The patients were as likely to be politically radical as the doctors. At the age of twenty, Alexander Bergman spent three weeks in the Bedford Sanitarium. In spite of faithful follow-up visits to an outpatient clinic, four years later he was admitted to Montefiore's South Pavilion with other advanced cases, "undernourished and emaciated." Pneumothorax was attempted.

Bergman, never to leave the hospital, devoted the rest of his short life to politics and poetry. One of his closest friends went off to fight in Spain and was killed. That struggle and the gathering war clouds all over Europe, together with the experiences of being a patient, were the subjects of his verse. On a spring day in 1941, he turned his face toward the light that came through the doorway and died, still believing that the hope of the world lay with Joseph Stalin. Only once had he received any money for a poem, $6.50 that *Poetry* had paid him for "April 29th," which dealt with the attack on Guernica. At his death, he left behind $13 and instructions that any future earnings from his verse should be divided equally between his family and *New Masses*.

Children were still an important part of life at Montefiore although the hospital still had no pediatric service. They came from the neighborhood schools to the cardiology clinic. Many of them were sent to the Mack Memorial Farm for the summer, and the sickest were admitted as inpatients, usually to die, for there was little that doctors could do to help hearts damaged by birth defects or the ravages of rheumatic fever except for the good food and fresh air of the summer vacations.

Not all the children died. R.S. was a normal, healthy baby and toddler. He came to Montefiore when the symptoms of cerebral palsy showed up after he started school. With halting speech and a clumsy walk, he was first taken to the Vanderbilt Clinic and then to the Neurological Division at Montefiore. Suspecting some form of lead poisoning, the doctors were unable to narrow the diagnosis further or to offer any treatment. In the meantime, the little boy's parents separated and he was left at Montefiore, which, according to him, became his "home, mother, and school."

He stayed for ten years, learning in Rose Woods' classroom, becoming a member of the boys' club, and since he didn't have to stay in bed, a happy messenger and errand boy for everybody in the Hospital. Busy and active, he saw the other children sick and pale. He knew that they died. All the children knew when one of them was dying because that child was taken out of the big ward to a single room. Running around the wards and corridors, R.S. thought of himself as strong and healthy.

He came out from behind the green iron fence a young man, old enough to join the Army and bitterly disappointed when he was rejected. He had not thought of himself as handicapped. Adjustment to the outside world was painful. Nevertheless, his strong self-image enabled him to go on to a career, marriage, and fatherhood.

The Jews who fled from Tsarist Russia escaped into a world that knew little of passports or visas. Most people traveled without any kind of official sanction. Those able to liberate themselves from poverty or pogrom entered the golden door without papers. In response to the floods of refugees released by World War I and the Depression, the nations of the world erected paper barriers as they sought to protect their own shaky economies by excluding aliens. Quotas and visas barred the way everywhere. Refugees from Hitler's Germany found doors closed. The rest of the world did not want them. They waited in the Channel ports. They haunted the consulates of every European city. The British turned them back from Palestine. The United States took a minuscule number and excluded the rest with careless brutality.

The Jewish community in the United States was not sure what action to take, unable to imagine the full extent of the horror, uncertain of its own acceptance in the wider society. Bluestone continued his efforts on behalf of refugee physicians —as did Boas. The Board was more wary, but there was no doubt of their patriotism toward the United States.

Montefiore became involved in World War II at an early

date. A month after the invasion of Poland and the outbreak of hostilities in Europe, the Board of Trustees placed the facilities of the Hospital at the disposal of the United States Government, promising that "in the emergency military program which our Government has undertaken Montefiore Hospital is willing and eager to play a part." The War Department thanked the Trustees and placed the correspondence "in a special classified mobilization file" until such time as the Department found itself in need of beds in the New York City area. The next spring, "an emergency operating set" was donated by the medical staff to the "Medical and Surgical Supply Committee of America to aid Great Britain and her Allies," ten members of the visiting staff were granted leave to go on active duty as commissioned officers, and patients and employees were busy collecting empty cigarette packages in order to take advantage of an offer by the cigarette companies "to send the Free French soldiers in Africa a full pack for every twenty empties collected." The lawn to the east of the Nurses' Residence was dug up for Victory gardens planted by the Parents' Association of P.S. 94.

The *Echo* announced that twenty-five graduates of the dietitian's courses held at Montefiore were now serving in the armed forces—all of them women, all of them lieutenants. Each issue of the paper carried names and addresses of former staff members now at war and the letters that came in regularly from Australia, India, and Europe. Dr. Adele B. Cohn (resident staff 1938–41), who went to China in 1941 for the American Bureau for Medical Aid to China, became assistant professor at the National Shanghai Medical College. Occasionally, there were announcements of death. Leo M. Friedman, public relations executive at Montefiore from 1940 to 1942, was seriously wounded while leading his platoon on an advanced sector on the Italian front and died a few days later. The *Echo* listed the Trustees who were "enrolled in the war effort and . . . on military leave of absence." One member of the Board was killed: Lieutenant Peter Gerald Lehman, oldest son of Herbert Lehman, who had succeeded Franklin D. Roosevelt as governor of New York.

The Board of Trustees organized a Defense Committee,

which met at the Harmonie Club in Manhattan. Dr. Sol Biloon was appointed as the Montefiore representative to the Bronx Defense Council and the decision was made that "the Country Sanitarium will be notified by the city institution in the event that an official alarm is received via the Army buzzer signal system." Two practice drills were held by the Montefiore "catastrophe squads," using students from Evander Childs High School as casualties.

While the Board was so actively concerned with the defense posture of the Hospital, some other aspects of the effect of the situation in Europe were not as close to their hearts as air-raid drills on Gun Hill Road. At the Board meeting held February 19, 1942, there was "some discussion as to the status of refugee applicants for appointments to our visiting staff. The original position of the Board concerning such refugees was reaffirmed (Americans to be preferred if other things are equal)."

The greatest immediate impact of the war on Montefiore was on the labor supply. Even before the United States entered the conflict in December 1941, a booming war industry and the expansion of the armed forces brought an end to the chronic unemployment that had persisted since the beginning of the Depression in spite of all of Roosevelt's efforts to prime the pump. Hospitals had been able, through all those years of high unemployment and low wages, to draw on a pool of cheap labor. The pool began to dry up quite rapidly.

More than seventy of the staff of visiting physicians joined the armed forces, more than a few of them in search of a steadier income than their Depression-ridden practices had afforded. Nurses enlisted for the same mixture of practicality and patriotism or found better-paying jobs in industry. The factories were desperate for workers, and groups such as women and blacks who had formerly been excluded found themselves welcome on the assembly lines. Montefiore found itself short of doctors, nurses, aides, orderlies, and kitchen help.

The Sanitarium lost 60 percent of its nursing staff; girls were brought in from the countryside roundabout and trained to do simple nursing chores. Since they were inexperienced, more of them had to be hired than normal and accommodations became a problem. Some of the healthier patients were asked to help out with the nursing as their contribution to the war effort.

The Hospital on Gun Hill Road was equally affected. The general shortage of employees encouraged those who remained to make demands for improvements in their working conditions. Some asked for a living-out allowance so that they could live away from the Hospital. The Board agreed to extend that privilege to ten or fifteen people, but resisted a request that overtime be paid at time and a half. Rosa Carlebach, the Trustee who chaired the Nursing Committee, at the first Board meeting held after Pearl Harbor reported that Montefiore had a shortage of twenty-one graduate nurses as well as a shortfall of seven male and female attendants. In the next breath she reported on a revolution that was taking place in nursing in New York City under the influence of the war-induced shortage. Until this time, black nurses could find employment in only one hospital in the Bronx, Lincoln, founded before the Civil War as "A Society for the Relief of Worthy, Aged, Indigent Colored Persons." Now Carlebach reported that Montefiore had twenty "colored" nurses, ten day and ten night. She said that they were "competent and working out successfully" but expressed doubts about the advisability of hiring any more.

The war years brought a constant struggle for the Hospital to survive and to provide patient care in spite of critical staff shortages. On one day in September 1943, there were 40 graduate nurses on duty instead of 54, 13 male attendants instead of 35, 28 female attendants instead of 44, and 5 ward maids instead of 14. Of these, 6 of the graduate nurses and 6 female attendants were not regular employees but temporaries hired from agencies.

Patient care was affected. One administrator reported: "These nurses are giving our patients a bare minimum of nursing care, but that minimum which can be given and still be consistent with good nursing care seems to grow ever smaller. . . . For example, a few Sundays ago, for the first time in the memory of any of our supervisors, beds were not stripped before being made; they were made, that is, by straightening the sheets, tightening the draw-sheets, and smoothing the pillowcases rather than by removing all linen and then replacing it."

Other kinds of care were curtailed: "Important medications are given as frequently as prescribed, even though not at the scheduled times. Vitamin capsules, aspirin tablets, and placebos of various sorts (which are still being ordered by the physicians) are occasionally overlooked, sometimes without the permission of the doctor or supervisor. Temperatures are now taken only when indicated; the nurses have been unable to comply with the ruling of the National Tuberculosis Association that daily temperatures be recorded on all tuberculous patients; at the very least, however, they are taken at least once every other day."

Some lapses were more keenly felt by the patients: "All too often patients must wait over-long for their bed pans to be brought, and then even longer for them to be taken away. This may account for a few of the many cases of incontinence in the Hospital."

Everybody realized that the problems were war-connected and tried to help: "The physicians have begun once more to do many of the surgical dressings which had been relegated to the nursing staff earlier in the year. . . . The physicians have learned to do many types of treatments without help and these include pneumothorax administration, intravenous infusions, transfusions, and wound irrigations."

For the first time, the Hospital set up an organized Volunteer Department, under the direction of Mrs. Lucille Isaac. While one group met regularly to make surgical dressings, another was recruited to train as lab technicians. This activity, according to Mrs. Isaac, did "not run smoothly because of lack of equipment and forgetfulness on the part of some doctors to leave instructions of work to be done."

Isaac's biggest problem, however, was the recruiting and training of nurse's aides. As she explained: "The week war broke out, I went to see Mrs. William Rotholz at the Red Cross. She is Regional Chief of all Red Cross Volunteer Nursing activities. I asked her to send us a Red Cross instructor. She said none was available for two months. She would not let us admit foreigners to the class. Would not allow women over 30. Would not promise to let us keep for our own use pupils trained at Montefiore."

Isaacs was not about to be defeated by the Red Cross. Other members of the Auxiliary rallied around and she was able to report: "Mrs. Warner Prins of our Women's Auxiliary gave a tea at her home to interest foreign women. I spoke to them and about ten signed up as Nurse's Aides. We started our own class with these women, plus many Bronx housewives—28 in all."

The volunteer program grew rapidly. In addition to the technicians and nurse's aides, there were others who fed patients unable to help themselves or worked in the Physiotherapy Department and the Patient's Library. Soon there was a roster of 400 volunteers ready to serve, including high school students and Boy Scouts, but they could not make up for the lack of full-time trained people.

Attempts were made to deal with staff shortages by discontinuing services. The children's wards were closed, as well as the Mack Memorial "temporarily." The children's cardiac clinic remained open.

In the winter of 1942–43, Bluestone, Moses, and other members of the Board met three times with representatives of Federation "to explain . . . the administrative difficulties that Montefiore found itself in because of the effects of the war . . . and to consult with them in regard to the only proposal that the Montefiore Trustees could see for lightening the load, namely the closing of the Schiff Pavilion, which still housed the custodial patients, provided the consent of Mrs. Warburg (Jacob Schiff's daughter) was given, and the patients could be properly placed."

The Social Service Department had already made a survey of the Schiff patients ("without, however," according to Moses, "consulting the patients or their families") and decided that fifteen of them could be moved to the main hospital, twenty-two could be returned to their own homes, some with a financial subsidy, a few could be sent to nursing homes with a subsidy, eight to homes for the aged, thirty-eight to homes for chronic invalids, and twenty-five to the new municipal hospital for the chronically ill, the Goldwater Memorial on Welfare Island. The Montefiore representatives emphasized that they had come to the meeting to discuss, not the financial problem, but the "public relations and communal questions involved."

There were lengthy discussions, not just about the Schiff Pavilion, but also about the difficult staffing problems faced by all the Federation hospitals. No alternative solution was found, and Federation agreed to the closing of the Schiff Pavilion, with it "clearly understood that Federation could not publicly take the lead in the matter, but would give whatever assistance was possible."

On January 16, having learned that Mrs. Warburg's health was too frail to permit of a meeting, Moses wrote to her son, describing the situation at great length and explaining all the measures taken to find more staff, even to the point that "about a year ago we were forced to adopt what was considered a very radical step, namely, employ colored graduate nurses, and at the present time, one third of our graduate nurses are colored."

Four days later, the Board voted to close the Schiff Pavilion. The plan devised by the Social Service Department was followed, sometimes with unexpected results. At the February Board meeting, Bluestone and Moses reported that one third of the patients had left and that "of this number one third had either returned to their homes or accepted employment elsewhere on a full-time basis."

Bluestone was a man of firm principles, ever ready to take advantage of opportunities to implement his own agenda. For more than ten years, he had been actively helping refugee physicians from Europe. The house staff shortage presented him with another chance to pursue two goals—assistance to refugees and more physicians on salary. He persuaded the Board that the only way to see that patients received adequate medical care was to hire paid assistants to chiefs of the various clinical divisions. The first four hired were all European refugees: Drs. Zalman Plotkin, Adolph D. Jonas, Frederick D. Stern, and George C. Leiner. Each was paid $200 a month with maintenance.

Competition for those residents who were not in the armed forces raised salaries. Assistant residents were now paid $50 a month instead of $25. Max Pinner, Chief of Pulmonary Services, asked for $1,500 as a temporary annual appropriation to subsidize his staff: the shortage impelled him to pay his physicians "$5.00 per morning, which is the equivalent paid by the Department of Health in its tuberculosis clinics."

Small raises were also given to the nurses, and another partial answer to the staffing problem was found, in an institution that already existed in embryo form. Two years before, New York State had brought another kind of nursing school to Montefiore when the legislature passed a law requiring that all persons professionally engaged in the care of the sick must be trained and licensed. Because there were so many patients who could not move themselves, Montefiore had always employed a number of male orderlies without any formal training to help lift and turn those too heavy or difficult for the nurses to manage. These were the positions most affected by the new law, and on April 1, 1940, the Montefiore School of Practical Nursing for Men opened with eight students enrolled for the nine-month course.

Faced with the nursing emergency, Bluestone and the Board decided to use the school to attract and train a new supply of nurses. With the approval of Albany, the School of Practical Nursing was expanded to work in collaboration with Bronx Hospital. Over the years of its existence, scores of black women passed through the courses and on to careers at Montefiore, at other hospitals, in the Visiting Nurse Service, and other fields. Many of them went on to become registered nurses. By December 1944, twenty-five students had been capped, in the traditional graduation ceremony for nursing schools. In the following month, thirty-three students began the course.

At the same time that Montefiore was struggling with a continuing staff shortage, the Hospital was admitting patients in need of more intensive care. The average patient was a much more acutely ill person. For the general public, Montefiore was a forbidding, frightening place where people came to die. This perception was not entirely untrue. Compared to that in general hospitals, the death rate was high: in 1942, 35 percent of all admissions. At Post-Graduate Hospital the same year, the death rate was 2.5 percent.

During the war years the mortality rate increased, 9 percent between 1939 and 1942. This may have been connected with the decrease in nursing care. More probably, however, the cause lay in the fact that patients came into the Hospital much sicker. In 1942, the waiting list disappeared, except in tuberculosis. Changes in medical care meant that many patients with chronic diseases, while not cured, no longer needed constant hospital care. Diabetics took their insulin home with them; diuretics enabled many heart patients to live at home. They came back to Montefiore, as did A., the female diabetic, when they were very sick, or beyond help and ready to die. Montefiore was changing into a different kind of a hospital.

13

Medicine on the Move

In spite of staff shortages, the pace of medical change quick-ened. In 1941, Lichtwitz's approaching retirement faced Bluestone with the need for a new Chief of Medicine. He found a man who would be one of the most influential figures in the history of Montefiore—Louis Leiter, who was to take an active part in the transformation of the Hospital for Chronic Diseases into an acute-care general hospital offering the most complex services.

The discovery of this physician was somewhat accidental. Two of Bluestone's nephews, both in medical school, happened to visit while he was casting about and told him that Louis Leiter, a nationally known nephrologist and head of the Section on Renal and Vascular Diseases at the University of Chicago, was not likely to achieve his hoped-for promotion to department chairman because he was Jewish.

Louis Leiter was born in Rumania and emigrated with his family to Montreal. He went to McGill and then to the University of Chicago and Rush Medical College, accumulating a Ph.D. and an M.D. From 1924 to 1926, he worked at the hospital of the Rockefeller Institute. He then spent a year in Vienna, Munich, and Hamburg before returning to Chicago and achieving a national reputation with his papers on kidney function.

Dr. Leiter's salary as the new Chief of the Medical Division was set at $10,000, with the understanding that (in lieu of a rent allowance) he could retain $1,200 a year of the fees paid to him by private patients. The balance of any money he earned would come to the Hospital. Dr. Lichtwitz was granted a bonus of six months' salary on his retirement.

The occasion of Lichtwitz's retirement party gave rise to one of the great Montefiore scandals, an event discussed in hushed tones for years afterward. All the resentments of the proud German doctor boiled over, all of the loneliness of exile, all the anger at the young men who didn't stand up when their chief came into the room, the frustrations with the lack of discipline, the hurt of the professional physician dependent on the whims of rich men for employment. As Moses reported: "Although Dr. Lichtwitz had stipulated that there was to be no speech-making, he himself addressed an audience of two hundred who had come to honor him, taking the occasion to denounce American hospitals generally as compared with German hospitals, and Montefiore Hospital in particular . . . the audience was shocked and mortified over this performance and . . . several of those present suggested that the appointment of Dr. Lichtwitz as consulting physician to our Hospital be rescinded." The Board moved immediately: "the decision to cancel the appointment of Dr. Lichtwitz and relieve him of any further association with the Hospital was made by unanimous vote." The announcement was made on the front page of the next edition of the *Echo* in a box outlined in black.

Leiter was a very different man from Lichtwitz, gentle and diffident, inspiring awe, not because of his manner, but by his intellectual attainments. Many a studious resident, struggling to stay awake in the library, was overcome by the sight of his chief, standing on one foot by the periodical shelves, riffling through the pages of a publication and apparently absorbing all the news of the latest research in a hasty glance. Each night he carried home with him a briefcase full of journals, feeling that, as chief, he had a duty to keep up with all the latest research. No Prussian aristocrat, a product of the educational system of the New World, he was yet no easy democrat, never taking kindly to advice from residents about how he should run his department. His manner tended to the aloof and formal. Jack Grossman, who knew him well and worked closely with him for almost forty years, described his resident's-eye view: "At first he impressed me as being somewhat austere, even stern at times. . . . It took me some time before I realized that some of his seeming aloofness was a need to preserve some degree of privacy."

Oppenheimer and Lichtwitz had ruled imperiously. Even their admirers had no desire to emulate their manners. Leiter inspired in many an ambition to be like him, to develop a bed-side demeanor as courteous and caring, and as probing. The residents who followed him on rounds saw a different kind of teaching and a different way of dealing with the patients in the long wards. He was incapable of treating any human being as "teaching material" or a "museum piece," of talking over people in bed as if they were deaf. The conversation with the patient did not consist of mere pleasantries. He was always trying to obtain more information, another piece of the puzzle.

Leiter was especially interested in kidney excretions. The body fluids and their chemical constituents could be accurately measured. Leiter combined within himself that concern for people and for science that is the best medicine, and he acted out his beliefs in a way that was visible to his students. Not all of his actions were so open. Those who were critical of him usually centered their discontent on a lack of action. He was accused more often of sins of omission than of commission, for not taking some vigorous step advocated by others. Sometimes appearances were deceptive, as Grossman found: "There was the feeling among the staff that Dr. Leiter's quiet demeanor, modesty, almost self-effacement, was of very little help in the advancement of his colleagues, research fellows or associates,

and there was an underlying criticism of his failure perhaps to
do more for some of his associates. I confess that it was a belief
that at one time I shared. Not until many years later did I
become aware of his attempts to help me in my own progress:
letters that were written for me, unknown to me, by Dr. Leiter
—letters which, when I read them much later, were very
moving."

His reputation attracted applications for internships and
residencies. The former he discouraged, feeling that a young
graduate fresh from medical school could learn more about the
profession in the hectic pace of the emergency room and wards
of an acute-care hospital. On the other hand, he saw a residency
at Montefiore as a superb way to specialize, to learn the long
and intricate course of heart disease or diabetes or kidney failure. Observing the slow degeneration, or the moments of re-
prieve, in the same patients day after day, month after month,
enabled the serious student to become totally familiar with the
face of the enemy, the ever-changing patterns of human
suffering.

Many hospitals in the United States were first forced to accept women as interns and residents when the men went off to
World War II. Montefiore continued its old tradition, and in the
war years several women who also played important roles in the
Hospital for many years joined the staff. Dr. Doris Escher arrived, to join the band of brilliant people involved in cardiology,
developing cardiac catheterization from an experimental procedure to a mainstay of diagnosis.

Shirley Grossman was accepted as an intern. "As soon as I
came in, I liked the place," she said. "I worked in Pathology and
I think that was a tremendously impressive experience, because
Dr. Marine was the Chief of Pathology and he was a very
famous man. He felt that the young house staff were his responsibility and it was his job to see that they were taken care
of." Grossman was not only a physician at Montefiore but a
patient. She came down with tuberculosis and spent months at
the Sanitarium. The experience became an important part of
learning how to be a caring physician.

Bluestone's view of medicine was all-inclusive. Part of his plan for the postwar period was to make Montefiore a center for psychiatry: "We feel that mental disease is as much entitled to the interest of the modern hospital as any other physical disease. . . . We are planning a 200-bed Institute of Neuropsychiatry to be erected on available Montefiore ground on Gun Hill Road."

Henry Moses shared this view. In 1942, the name of the division was changed from Neurology to Neuropsychiatry, and two years later the two men, in a great coup, persuaded Houston Merritt to leave Harvard and come to Montefiore. Merritt had achieved fame and enormous impact on the field of neurology by discovering, with his co-worker Tracy Putnam, a specific drug treatment for epilepsy, one of the commonest of neurological disorders. The only effective drug used in epilepsy until that time was phenobarbitol, which was a sedative and therefore made it impossible for the patient to function normally while under treatment. In research on animals, Merritt and Putnam developed Dilantin (diphenylhydantoin), which became and remains probably the most widely used anti-seizure drug in the world. Merritt also made important contributions to an understanding of exactly how syphilis affects the brain, and he and his colleagues accurately measured the fluid that surrounds the brain and spinal cord, showing the relationship between various abnormalities and particular disorders.

Before his retirement, Marine took part with Leiter and others in an experiment that was a step into a different kind of therapy. All the years of thyroid research at Montefiore came together in the early forties with the beginning of nuclear medicine. One patient, B., originally suffered from goiter. In 1923, after an operation performed to remove his thyroid, the tissue was found to be cancerous. For about fifteen years after the operation, B. appeared healthy. Then, in 1938, he developed the symptoms of hyperthyroidism—a sudden loss of weight and extreme nervousness. Along with these signs, totally surprising in someone not in possession of a thyroid gland, B. had severe constant pain in his lower back and radiating down his legs. Doctors (at another hospital) found a tumor in the middle of his back. The tumor was removed and found to be a metastatic thyroid carcinoma. After that operation, the patient's symptoms of hyperthyroidism, instead of decreasing, increased. X-rays showed metastatic deposits in both lungs and some destruction of the right upper femur and the second left rib, the growths acting as if they themselves were glands, sending thyroid secretions out through B.'s body.

B. arrived at Montefiore in April 1942, "a rather small, emaciated, poorly developed individual, aged 48." A constellation of people profoundly knowledgeable about the thyroid gathered around B., including Sam Seidlin, an endocrinologist whom Leiter had brought to Montefiore. Seidlin found that some radioactive iodine was available as a by-product of atomic research, and the physicians decided to use radioactive iodine as a tracer.

Seidlin obtained the radioiodine from a contact in St. Louis. Since all the separate metastases scattered over B.'s body seemed to be acting as if they themselves were thyroid glands, there was a possibility that they would attract iodine in the same way that the thyroid absorbs the substance. B. was fed radioactive sodium iodine in water. Geiger counter measurement showed iodine retention by all the known lesions plus two previously unsuspected. The diagnosis was followed by therapy. B. continued to receive doses of the same medication, which began to affect the lesions. He improved. The thyroid activity slowed down, he put on weight and was able to get out of bed, wander around the hospital, and even to go home for weekends.

B.'s case was not only the impetus for the development of the radioisotope program at Montefiore but also the subject of many papers. Together with two of his collaborators, L. D. Marinelli and Eleanor Oshry, Seidlin published a paper, "Radioactive Iodine Therapy," which appeared in the *Journal of the American Medical Association* on December 7, 1946. Seidlin thanked all the people at Montefiore who had helped: "Dr. Louis Leiter, Chief of the Medical Division of Montefiore Hospital, gave valuable assistance throughout this work, as did Dr. David Marine and Dr. S. H. Rosen in the field of thyroid pathology and Dr. E. J. Baumann in iodine chemistry. Dr. Solomon Fineman reviewed the roentgenograms. Valuable technical assistance was rendered by Elizabeth F. Focht, Ruth Hill, George Ross, Louella Tulip and Dr. A. A. Yalow." Dr. Yalow's wife, Rosalyn, who was to return to Montefiore as a Nobel laureate and Chairman of Clinical Sciences, assisted as a volunteer, implementing the method that Baumann had devised for retrieving the expensive isotopes from the patient's urine.

In the meantime, Marine had retired, still as careful of other people's money as ever. By 1929, his salary had risen to $12,000. He loved to spend his summers on the Delaware shore and asked to take a cut in salary so that he could enjoy a long vacation. As a result, in 1932 his salary went back to $10,000, where it remained until his retirement in 1945, at which time the Board of Trustees awarded him the rank of consulting pathologist and the sum of $12,000, "to be paid to him at his discretion in a lump sum or in one or more annual payments." Marine refused to accept the money.

The new Chief of Pathology at Montefiore was Harry Zimmerman. His greatest contributions came in the field of neuropathology, but when he was a resident at Yale Medical School in the twenties there was not a single full-time department or division devoted to the subject in any medical school in the United States. When Dean Winternitz, chairman of the Department of Pathology at Yale, decided that his students needed an instructor in neuropathology, there was no one qualified to teach the topic. Winternitz decided that one of his residents should be trained for the job, and in 1929 provided Zimmerman with a traveling fellowship to study abroad.

Zimmerman returned to Yale to set up a section of neuropathology within the Department of Pathology. His neuropathological section flourished in an atmosphere of collaborative research. Zimmerman also worked with the Department of Physiological Chemistry on studies of the effect of vitamin deficiencies—beriberi, pellagra, xerophthalmia, and hypervitaminosis D. At the same time, the neuropathological section was concerned with the effect of chemical carcinogens on the brain.

Many had assumed that Zimmerman would succeed Win-

ternitz in the chair at Yale. Passed over, Zimmerman accepted
the position of Chief of the Laboratory Division at Montefiore
when David Marine retired.

At Montefiore, Dr. Harry Zimmerman continued working
with Sam Seidlin on the mysteries of the thyroid: "When I arrived in 1946, I quickly learned that Dr. Seidlin not only was
interested in those aspects that have already been mentioned,
but he wanted strict scientific control. I got involved because I
was the pathologist and he insisted on my diagnosing the biopsies of the thyroid gland which he removed first from this
well-known patient, on whom he made the original observation
of the iodine uptake of the thyroid tumor, and on all subsequent
patients. Then he would persuade these patients to permit
needle and open biopsies of the thyroid gland to see whether the
effect of radioactive iodine really was ablating the tumor or
changing the morphological characteristics."

The third member of the triumvirate arrived in the difficult
persona of Leo Davidoff. According to his own account, he was
"the greatest Jewish neurosurgeon," and he was probably right.
He studied under Harvey Cushing (and was determined in his
own teaching service to emulate the great man) and all his life
pursued perfection, to the distress of many a hospital administrator. In brain surgery the odds against success were always
astronomical, and Davidoff struggled to give his patients every
chance possible. He did his own dressings; he tried out every
new method for ensuring total sterility in his operating room.
His residents were expected to meet his high standards at all
times: absolute punctuality on rounds and complete preparation
in the operating room.

Davidoff made demands at Montefiore. With the income he
brought into the Hospital amounting to $100,000 a year, and
his salary fixed at $25,000, he asked for a larger slice of the pie.
In April 1946, he asked for a three-month leave of absence to
teach in Prague. The leave was granted, and in a conference
with the Medical Committee, Davidoff promised to "integrate
his work with that of the Hospital and devote more time to ward
work." In return, the money he brought in was to be divided

equally between himself and the Hospital, his life insurance was to be paid by the Hospital, and he was to be given $10,000 a year for research.

One of the great disappointments of the postwar years was that the Neuropsychiatric Institute was never built. The move to Montefiore had guaranteed Merritt a place on the faculty at Columbia, and in 1948 he left Montefiore to become chairman of the Department of Neurology at Columbia and director of the neurological section of the Neurological Institute of Presbyterian Hospital. (This was the only occasion during the long years of the Montefiore-Columbia connection that one of the Montefiore people who had a faculty appointment at Columbia was promoted to a chairmanship at Columbia. Of course, almost all of the others were Jewish.)

Davidoff had a stormy on-and-off relationship with Montefiore, resigning and returning. He left Bluestone but came back under his successor, who when a Board member asked how he managed to get along with Davidoff, explained that he just gave the surgeon everything he wanted. Zimmerman stayed on to become one of the builders of the new Montefiore—and, with Davidoff, of that Jewish medical school of which so many had dreamed.

The death rate from tuberculosis fell all during the twentieth century, from 194.4 per thousand in 1900 to 55.1 in 1935 to 39.9 in 1945. The likelihood is that it was also falling during the nineteenth century as the general level of nutrition and housing improved. New York City, overcrowded, with a constant incoming supply of poverty-stricken immigrants, usually had a higher rate than healthier sections of the country. To sort out the relative importance of the various factors involved is impossible: better food, better housing, better sanitation, public awareness of the mechanisms of infection, the sanitarium movement, earlier diagnosis with X-rays, specific methods of treatment such as the collapsing of lungs. What is clear is that the introduction of drug therapy produced a sudden rapid drop in the mortality rate.

Streptomycin, isolated by Selman A. Waksman in 1944, was

the third of the wonder drugs, following the sulfas and penicillin. Before the end of the year a test began on a young woman with severe, far advanced tuberculosis. Treatment was complicated. There were impurities in the drug, and no one was sure of what the side effects might be or what the safe dosage was. The experiment was successful, but it was not until twenty months after she started on the drug that the patient was able to leave the hospital. Waksman and Rutgers University turned over control of the drug to Merck and Company for the extended testing that took place in hospitals in Great Britain and the United States. The success of previous wonder drugs had raised the expectations of professionals and public.

Quickly it became clear that streptomycin was effective against tuberculosis affecting most parts of the body: lungs, bones, joints, genitourinary organs, and skin. Montefiore was invited to participate in the early tests. The Division of Pulmonary Diseases (under Eli Rubin) and the Laboratory Division (under Harry Zimmerman) used the drug on thirty-one patients, most of them from the Sanitarium, from October 1946 to mid-June 1947. They were all people whose condition was deteriorating in spite of prolonged bed rest and, in some cases, lung collapse. After that forty-four even more seriously ill patients were treated with crystalline streptomycin. Many in this second group were desperately ill, "the streptomycin being given more in the hope than in the expectation of obtaining any benefit." Eight had diabetes as well as tuberculosis. One was a four-year-old child with meningeal tuberculosis. One had advanced tuberculosis, laryngitis, and asthma.

Only one patient did not show improvement, and a few suffered no side effects at all. About half developed persistent dizziness, dermatitis, occasional vomiting, headache, or stomatitis (inflammation of the mouth). In a few, reactions were severe enough to stop treatment. The patients were so anxious for treatment that they often lied about any discomfort and begged the doctors to continue in spite of side effects or the pain of the injections, which went on for months every four hours, day and night.

This was the beginning of a revolution, but the Montefiore physicians were cautious in their assessment: "In the present state of knowledge of the value and limitations of streptomycin, it is inadvisable to use the agent as a shortcut in the treatment of pulmonary tuberculosis or, for that matter, as a routine method of treatment under any circumstance. As long as there is a reasonable expectation of obtaining arrest of the disease on a modern sanitarium regimen, streptomycin should be reserved for special indications." In the long run tuberculosis was not to be controlled by one drug. Strains of bacteria resistant to streptomycin appeared. The future lay with combinations of drugs.

At the same time that these first steps leading to the control of tuberculosis were underway, cases of the other great disease of the lungs were increasing rapidly: during the forties the number of deaths from lung cancer were up more than 50 percent, most of the victims men. In the twenties Maurice Fishberg attributed the rise in lung cancer to the flu epidemic of 1917. Dr. Milton B. Rosenblatt, an attending physician in the Division of Pulmonary Diseases, was still not ready to accept smoking as the culprit, writing in 1949: "The tremendous increase in the incidence of bronchogenic carcinoma has been attributed to carcinogenic influences such as tobacco and tarring of roads. Most observers, however, feel that the increase is due mainly to (I) improved methods of diagnosis and (II) the increase in population reaching late adult life. Analysis of the statistics reveals that the increase in cancer has occurred chiefly in the older age groups."

The wonder drugs affected the pattern of other diseases at Montefiore. Penicillin was used against syphilis as early as 1943. The national death rate from that disease was halved between 1940 and 1950 and halved again by 1955. The drug was useful against old as well as new cases. Many of both the adults and children at Montefiore with heart conditions had been damaged by rheumatic fever. The illness usually began with the symptoms of scarlet fever or a sore throat caused by a streptococcal infection, followed by red, swollen, painful joints. Often the heart muscle was affected so that it could not pump strongly enough or the valves of the heart became misshapen or an envelope of scar tissue grew around the heart so that it could not expand fully. As doctors began to treat scarlet fever and sore throats with penicillin, fewer and fewer cases of rheumatic fever and its aftereffects were seen.

The sulfa drugs, streptomycin, and penicillin fundamentally changed the practice of medicine. A wide range of infectious diseases came under control, and the possibilities of surgery widened as the ability to deal with infection increased.

Hospitals lost the role that had, since medieval times, often been their most important function: isolating the infectious from their communities. At the same time, their importance as centers for surgery and diagnosis increased. The role of the drug companies in the structure of the health-care system was enhanced. They used their enormous profits to fund research products, and public and professionals alike now expected a constant stream of wonder drugs to flow from the laboratories.

CHAPTER

14

Brave New World

The United States came out of the war eager and restless
for change, with an unbounded faith in science and technology, in a hurry to grow, to expand, and to create the perfect
life for all its citizens. The Montefiore Board, with several
members returned from military duty, approached the postwar
world with the same eagerness for change and growth. One of
the up-and-coming young members of the Board was George
Kirstein, brother of Lincoln Kirstein, the godfather of the New
York City Ballet. George shared the family's intellectual brilliance, adding a fierce concern for social issues. Already he was
Chairman of the Committee for Post War Planning, and now
Moses made him chairman of a committee which was, among
other things, "to investigate various proposed expansion plans of
the Hospital, taking into consideration the additional amount of
space, personnel, and financing required in connection there-
with." In effect, the committee was to decide the future of the
Hospital, and it was headed by a lively young man, unsympathetic to Bluestone's measured dignity, however much he admired Bluestone's social vision and programs.

Moses was anxious to have the Trustees make more visits to the Hospital, and he appointed tough, dynamic Victor Riesenfeld to organize their visits, encouraging them to sit in on conferences between the President and the Director. The days of peace for Bluestone were over. Trustees and committees of the Board constantly visited the Hospital, prodding and prying and asking questions, and at times it must have seemed that they all consisted of George Kirstein or Victor Riesenfeld, who had been appointed chairman of a subcommittee "to consider the present financial operations together with the financial aspects of the construction and maintenance of additional projects in the postwar program." These were men who had devoted their lives to understanding finances. A man of Bluestone's indifference to money matters found them most uncomfortable.

There had been no major construction at Montefiore since the twenties, and the years of financial restriction, of depression and war, had taken their toll of the physical plant in inadequate maintenance and lack of modernization. The Trustees consulted with Edwin A. Salmon, Hospitals Commissioner of the City of New York, who agreed to work with the well-known architectural firm of Skidmore, Owings and Merrill to draw up designs based on Bluestone's programmatic plans. Matters proceeded slowly. Two years and seven months later, Salmon's final report was almost ready, and no actual building was completed until 1951, six years after that first rush of enthusiasm. The main feature of the Salmon plan, an eleven-story building costing $7 million, was never built.

By the end of 1945, Moses was expressing deep concern over the mounting deficit, which was approaching $200,000 a year. Almost all the patients were charity cases, costing $6.00 a day for maintenance. For those patients it subsidized, the city paid only $2.60 a day. Moses discussed the possibility of converting some wards for the use of paying patients as one solution, while Fred Stein recommended an increase in the private and semi-private rates.

Beds were empty at the Country Sanitarium, with the Veterans Administration taking care of many men with tuberculosis who might otherwise have come to Bedford.

Most alarming was the fact that there were so many empty beds, fifty-eight at the latest count at Montefiore, and no waiting list. Moses saw two reasons for the situation: families were earning enough money to be able to take care of their sick members at home and there was a greater interest in chronic disease on the part of acute-care institutions. A quarter of the beds at Montefiore were actually closed because of a lack of personnel, especially nurses.

In the spring of 1946, Victor Riesenfeld called the attention of the Board of Trustees—"sharply," according to the minutes—to the "serious" financial position of the Hospital, operating at a monthly deficit of $30,000. Riesenfeld predicted a budget deficit of $800,000 for the next year, pointing out that Montefiore's free funds were exhausted and that expenses in those inflationary postwar times were constantly rising.

Many different ways of raising money were explored. Until now outpatient services had been free. The Board decided to charge as much as $1.00 a visit in cases where the patient could afford the fee. Attempts were made to sell or lease Big Tree Farm. Rates in the Private Pavilion were raised: a bed in a semiprivate ward went up by 50 cents to $6.00 a day; for $7.00 one could have one of the two beds in a double room; for $12, the promise that the other bed would be left empty; $15 bought the double room with one bed occupied by the patient and the other by an attendant. The Medical Board suggested various ways of coping with the varying ability of patients to pay, recommending in 1946 that charges for anesthesia be set for ward patients at $5.00 for minor surgery and $10 for major, and that private patients be charged anything from $15 to $75 according to income. To assist the accounting department in making decisions, the operating surgeon was asked to note on the anesthesia chart "P" for poor, "M" for moderate, or "W" for wealthy.

For the first time, the Trustees thought in terms of the federal government subsidizing the teaching program: Bluestone was authorized "to execute papers in order to collect various sums from the Veterans Administration, for out-of-pocket money in connection with the training of medical veterans."

The end of the war did not solve the nursing shortages: women who had delayed marriage or families were concentrating their efforts on the postwar baby boom; others found more lucrative fields than hospital nursing open to them. Mrs. Carlebach reported for the Committee on Nursing that, as in the past, Montefiore's problems were aggravated by the distance from Manhattan and the lack of interest in caring for the chronically ill. In an attempt to hold on to the nurses then working, the committee authorized a raise of $25 for registered nurses and $10 for practical nurses.

To underline the gravity of the situation, an all-male emergency committee was appointed to assist Carlebach in "attempting to solve the nursing situation." The committee produced a report, the central theme of which was that Montefiore, to attract a sufficient number of nurses, would have to compete with working conditions at other hospitals. The city of New York and the Veterans Administration both offered a forty-hour workweek made up of eight-hour continuous shifts. The Board agreed to a similar pattern and voted the $50,000 necessary to pay for the extra coverage.

The Board ruminating about the future bore a strong resemblance to the Board of the past, concerned about such administrative details as the widening of elevator doors or the electrification of the dumbwaiter in the West Building. A new administrator found that all applications for admission were still passed on by the Board, one of his duties being to carry a sheaf of applications downtown on the subway to the offices or homes of members of the Board of Trustees.

The Board was not about to leap lightly into the twentieth century. At the October Board meeting in 1946, "Mr. Freudenthal recommended that the Hospital purchase a check signing machine in order to save the time of the check signing officers. There was an extended discussion as to the advisability of doing so. It was decided to take the matter up at the January meeting."

In the end, great changes, revolutionary changes, were brought about at Montefiore, not by the Board of Trustees, which so carefully planned and plotted the course, but by Bluestone, the man who never worried about finances or buildings. He succeeded in these postwar years in putting into practice some of his most cherished ideas.

The problems involved in releasing patients from Montefiore remained remarkably similar over the years. Cures were few. The Hospital was becoming more and more successful, however, in improving and stabilizing the patient's condition. High blood pressure was brought down and edema relieved. In diabetic patients insulin levels were controlled. In the arthritic and paralyzed wasted muscles were strengthened. Even cancer patients began to survive for longer periods of time. The patients could return home—if there was room, if there was continuing medical supervision, if some nursing care could be provided, if a suitable diet was possible.

Cancer patients were now part of the Medical Service. Leiter felt that they were being short-changed, that they, and the Hospital, would benefit from the special attention of an expert. That was not a popular idea at the time. A few special cancer hospitals were in existence. Most general hospitals did not have enough cancer patients or enough physicians interested in their hopeless cases to justify a separate service. Leiter felt differently. The man he brought to Gun Hill Road to head the Cancer Service was to be remembered for many of the same qualities as his Chief of Medicine: the rigorous mind of a scientist combined with sympathetic compassion for every patient. Their students learned the same lessons of heart and mind from both.

Daniel Laszlo, born in Kassa, Hungary, in 1903, received his medical degree from the University of Vienna and served with the Departments of Medicine in Freiberg and Cologne before returning to Vienna. He came from Europe to New York in the year of the Anschluss and joined the staff of the cancer research unit at Mount Sinai. This group studied substances that produced tumors in mice and developed some of the first chemotherapeutic agents. He was happy to leave the benches at Mount Sinai and devote himself to patients at Montefiore, giving them both a personal sympathy and an unrelenting intensity of medical care.

Bluestone's views about the appropriate use of hospital beds were always intense: "If the use of hospital facilities is restricted to those who require intensive scientific care, we shall find that more hospital beds are available for more people." When Laszlo and Leiter suggested sending some patients home, he responded.

Hospital care, he thought, was expensive, not only financially but also emotionally. Even the best of hospitals is an institution where the patient is deprived of the comfort of accustomed routines and surroundings, of the warmth of homely sounds and smells and flavors. The answer was to send the patient home: "The Home Care patient's bedroom becomes, in effect, a unit of the Hospital. Here, in familiar, friendly surroundings, he receives the same care that he would be given in the Hospital, administered by the same members of the Hospital treatment team—the staff physician, the consultant and specialists in his illness, the social service worker, the occupational therapist, the physical therapist and others."

Home Care began with the aim of providing for thirty to thirty-five patients at a time. During the first six months, the average number was twenty; in the next six months, forty. At first (since the money was provided by the New York City Cancer Committee) only cancer patients were considered. Soon a grant from the Greater New York Fund, with no restrictions as to the nature of the disease, allowed the inclusion of people with heart disease, peripheral vascular disease, neurological disturbances, diabetes, tuberculosis, arthritis, and ulcerative colitis. The following year, with a grant from the New York Heart Association, children with rheumatic heart disease were accepted as Home Care patients. The adults received medical care from physicians, nursing care from the Visiting Nurse Service, special services, physical and occupational therapy, and where necessary, help with housekeeping. All the backup services of the Hospital were available: the labs, pharmacy, X-rays, etc. Additionally, the children benefited from the services of a psychiatric social worker, a child psychiatrist, a nutritionist, psychological testing, and homebound instruction from the Board of Education.

Patients were carefully selected. During the first year, 240 were recommended for the program, but thirty-five were disapproved for medical reasons, thirty-two for "geographic reasons," twenty-three because of no available home, and twenty-nine because of "unsuitable home." Of those who were accepted for Home Care, forty were later readmitted to the Hospital, and of these, nineteen died. Fourteen patients were discharged to the Outpatient Department and nine discharged "in other ways." Thirteen died at home.

There were also the patients who traveled in the opposite direction. Within that first year there were two—one of whom had been at Montefiore for months, the other for years—who took their first steps at home. Many procedures were safely performed in the cluttered Bronx apartments: those blood transfusions which ten years before had seemed to Dr. Bluestone such expensive experiments (one patient had ten transfusions at home in two months), tappings of the abdomen to release accumulated fluid. During the year, in addition to the physicians who provided the day-to-day services, neurological surgeons, ophthalmologists, general surgeons, and orthopedists were called in.

Martin Cherkasky had returned to Montefiore after learning hospital administration in the Army. After a few months as a Fellow in Medicine catching up on a body of knowledge that had developed fast during the years of war, then ten months as Chief Resident, he was appointed by Bluestone as executive of the Home Care Department.

Bluestone was his usual cautious, controlled self, still watching from his office window to make sure that employees arrived on time. Martin Cherkasky was one of thousands of young men with families and a drive to make up for years spent in the Army. He was the perfect instrument for Bluestone. The older man was a theoretician, able to conceptualize programs that challenged the basic organization of medical care. The young man was able to put them into practice—and sell them to professionals and public. As Administrator of Home Care, he was also one of the visiting doctors, climbing the tenement steps, black bag in hand, learning about the realities of life and death in the Bronx from his patients and from the social workers with whom he made rounds.

Another of Bluestone's innovations reflected three of his basic beliefs: the importance of non-medical care as part of treatment, the role of the family in patient support, and the need for co-operation between physicians and social workers.

Visiting relatives at Montefiore was difficult for families. Visiting hours were limited. Unless they lived in the immediate neighborhood, distances were formidable—and Montefiore still drew patients from all over the city. Social workers were not usually available for questions on evenings or weekends. Few patients had private doctors ready to talk with families.

In August 1948, Bluestone started a new procedure. Tuesday evenings, immediately before the normal visiting hours, relatives were invited to come to the auditorium, where each family met with the resident and the social worker assigned to sick son, mother, or father. The family was encouraged to ask questions. Minna Field, the Social Service Executive, said that the most common questions were: What's wrong with the patient? What will the illness mean to our future family living? How much will the patient be able to do when he or she returns home?

The experience was valuable for the young residents, training them to deal with families, teaching them to translate medical jargon into understandable English, to say "outlook" instead of "prognosis," to say "infection" instead of "subacute bacterial endocarditis." They also learned to work with another professional, the social worker, trained in different skills and with a different store of useful knowledge. To a family preparing for the return home of a patient, the social worker was able to translate the physician's instructions about diet or lifestyle into suggestions appropriate for the family's ethnic background or economic circumstances.

The prospect of the patient's return home was not always welcome to a family. As in Boas' day, the economic or nursing burdens often appeared overwhelming. Doctor and social worker together helped the family overcome the barriers, with suggestions about other available resources, reassurance that Montefiore's services would always be accessible.

Exactly one year after the inception of Home Care, Bluestone's next experiment—the Montefiore Medical Group—opened its doors. Medical care, backed by the full facilities of the Hospital, was made accessible on a voluntary, prepaid basis to people earning less than $5,000 a year ($6,500 for a family) and enrolled in the Health Insurance Plan (HIP) of Greater New York.

Prepaid group practice was regarded, inside and outside the Hospital, with great suspicion, and Bluestone overcame widespread opposition to a scheme that was seen as an undermining of the traditional economic base of medical practice. Mayor Fiorello La Guardia, after studies showed that the high cost of health care was a principal reason for city employees to sink into hopeless debt, first described HIP in one of his regular Sunday afternoon radio broadcasts to the people of New York City in 1944. Five months later, eighty civic leaders, including Bluestone, were announced as official incorporators of the Plan. The Director of Montefiore still had to persuade his Board of Trustees of the validity of prepaid group medicine. Moses was enthusiastic; the Trustees were uneasy. At the beginning of 1946 a committee reported back to the Board:

1. That Montefiore Hospital was not under an obligation to be one of the leaders in such a plan.
2. That the medical staff of our Hospital had an adequate amount of clinical material and did not require more.
3. That the problem of space for the Clinic would probably be an unsurmountable obstacle . . .
4. That we would have to add to our medical staff to the extent of approximately twenty-five full- and part-time men.

Perhaps the most serious objection was "that the establishment of the Clinic would be the entrance of acute service 'thru the back door.'" Bluestone was not to be deterred. An expert consultant, Lieutenant Colonel Henry B. Makover of the United States Public Health Service, was hired to produce a study in response to the objections of the Board. Questions about finances were answered optimistically: "During the first year or two of operation, no profit could be confidently expected, but there is good reason to believe that a grant may be received to guarantee us for several years against a deficit. The capital investment for construction and equipment for the group clinic must be found, but if it can be shown that group practice will be profitable, a real incentive to philanthropy exists."

The problem of a supply of beds could be as easily solved: "If the hospitalization needs cannot be met by the use of the present private facilities, patients could be hospitalized in general hospitals in which the group's physicians have privileges."

By such arguments was the Board of Trustees won over and the Group went into operation. Philanthropy was still a major force at Montefiore, contributing a third of the budget. Henry Moses, at first the President of the Board of Trustees and then the head of the Committee on Social Medicine in these years, was in the mold of Jacob Schiff, wealthy, politically conservative, but concerned for the total well-being of patients, ready to provide money for the latest in medical equipment or for experiments in the delivery of health care. Moses helped to persuade the more reluctant Board members and contributed a large part of the $25,000 donation from the Board that, together with grants from the Josiah Macy, Jr., Fund and the Milbank Memorial Fund, a $27,000 loan from HIP, and $7,500 from David Heyman of the New York Foundation, made possible the start-up of the Medical Group at Montefiore.

Some physicians at Montefiore objected to the formation of the Group as an attack on the private practice of medicine, objecting even to the fact that the Group physicians were paged on the Montefiore system. Other physicians found a haven there. After her bout with tuberculosis, Shirley Grossman went back to Montefiore. "I had been out of work a year and a half, and it was very hard getting back when you stay in bed so long. Dr. Cherkasky gave me a job there for one hour a day. Then it went to two hours a day, and after a while I began to work full-time, and I stayed with the Group ever after."

Bluestone next began to think about a Division of Social Medicine for his hospital and also about another idea—the Peckham Experiment, a pioneer health center set up in London to provide preventive medical services, not just to individuals, but to families as units. As many as 1,500 families, each paying one shilling a week and varying in economic origin from poor to middle class, joined the program. Each family could make use of a wide range of services: "an ante-natal clinic, post-natal clinic, birth control clinic, infant welfare clinic, care of the toddler, nursery schools, immunization center, medical inspection of the school-child, vocational guidance, sex instruction of adolescents, boys' and girls' clubs, sports clubs, and recreational clubs of all kinds."

Bailey Burritt of the Community Service Society was interested in the Peckham Experiment as a way of improving the health of families. Martin Cherkasky was interested in extending and studying the impact of the care offered to families through the Medical Group, and was heavily involved in the discussions and negotiations that brought the Peckham idea to Montefiore as the Family Health Maintenance Demonstration. Sorting through the abundance of articles, studies, and proposals that the original center had provoked, and calling on the lessons he had learned as an administrator in war and peace, he was able to produce a plan practical for the time and place. The families and the medical staff came from the Montefiore Medical Group, and the money from the Community Service Society and the Milbank Fund. This experiment to judge the impact of long-term social and medical services on family life in the Bronx was conducted under the guidance of a governing board with members drawn from the Society, the Hospital, HIP, and the Columbia-Presbyterian Medical Center.

Bluestone, once he had appointed his usual director, went to the Board of Trustees to ask that the whole enterprise be put together as a Division of Social Medicine, which would also oversee the existing social services of the Hospital. The Board worried about the expense but was reassured by Bluestone's reminder of the $375,000 that foundations had given to the social medicine programs in the past three years. Cherkasky became full-time chief of the division with responsibility for social services, Home Care, the Medical Group, the Family Health Demonstration Center, social statistics, education and research in social medicine, and "cooperation with all other divisions and independent services of the hospital."

The patients enrolled in the Medical Group were not the chronically sick. They were young families whose medical problems usually required the facilities of an acute-care hospital: more operating rooms, more intensive nursing care, a wider range of medical specialties.

The construction planned by the Board allowed for a different kind of medicine than had been practiced in the past: $340,000 for repairs and rehabilitation and $650,000 for two one-story diagnostic and surgery buildings in the Hospital's central courtyards, with space for ten operating rooms, six X-ray rooms, recovery rooms, waiting rooms, and so on. (For many years, Montefiore had managed with two major operating rooms and one minor.)

The new operating rooms were to prove a powerful force propelling Montefiore along the road of change. Initially, they solved a problem: there were now enough operating rooms to avoid delays. The cost of running them was high and had to be covered by increased use by patients who were able to pay, usually through insurance of some kind. All in all, Montefiore was entering an era of dispensing a more expensive brand of medicine, beyond the capability of charity to subsidize.

The collection of money was complicated. Montefiore's funds no longer arrived principally in the form of large checks from individual philanthropy, Federation, the United Hospital Fund, or the city of New York. Each of these new patients had to be billed individually and the claims for reimbursement filed in accordance with Blue Cross or HIP regulations.

Montefiore had begun to move in the direction where the money was. In spite of his belief that it was his job to run the Hospital and the task of the Board of Trustees to worry about the money, Bluestone long ago had one astonishing insight into the economics of health care. Boas advocated special institutions for the care of the chronically ill. Bluestone disagreed—on financial grounds. He believed that the chronically ill needed the same highly scientific care and complex technology as the acutely ill. The slow turnover and the infrequency of use of the skilled people and the machines in a hospital for long-term illness could not justify the cost. Quite early in his professional career Bluestone decided that the only way the most expert care could be guaranteed for long-term patients was to house them in institutions that included short-term patients. His new programs had the effect of turning Montefiore toward becoming the kind of hospital of which he had always dreamed. Home Care took long-term patients out of the hospital; the Medical Group brought in short-term patients, and the funds to pay for them. For the first time in Montefiore's history there was a large number of private patients, able to pay their own way, not dependent on charity. These people were not rich. Their ability to meet their bills came from insurance.

Bluestone challenged the economic system of fee-for-service medicine, which so horrified the young man and which was the well-defended norm of American medicine. He did so for the best of reasons—the welfare of patients. He did so, however, with little understanding of economics or finances. Easily confused by mathematics, bored by budgets, he had small grasp of the financial implications of his proposals. Asked by a newly arrived administrative resident about the previous year's deficit, Bluestone denied that there had been a deficit. Confronted with the figures, he cheerfully remarked, "Oh, they must have forgotten to tell me about it." The days of such insouciance were disappearing. Health care was about to become big business. Financial innocence was as inappropriate in a hospital administrator as the Victorian manner. The time had come for a change in leadership.

In 1950, Bluestone resigned his post, and Cherkasky was appointed Director, assuming the leadership of an institution in the process of being reshaped by external and internal forces.

The lawyers and the accountants and the computer experts arrived, and they all called each other by their first names as they built the complex structure that is today's Montefiore on that interesting base designed by that very proper radical, Ephraim Michael Bluestone.

CHAPTER

15

The Power of Persuasion

W hen the Trustees, with Victor Riesenfeld at their head, appointed the new Director, they were not entirely clear about the role he was to play or the amount of authority he was to be allowed. Cherkasky later described the process: "In the first year, they were very uncertain because it was a big budget and a big job, but what did they know about whether I could run Montefiore? But after the first year, when Victor Riesenfeld came to the conclusion that I wasn't going to make a shambles of it, I had free rein."

During his leadership of Montefiore, hospitals, bolstered by money, technology, and public and private policy, became the central institutions in health care. Taking advantage of the times and of the resources increasingly available through public and quasi-public agencies, Cherkasky constructed, on the foundation of an institution for the care of long-term illness, a complex, powerful medical center. He also built on the concerns with families and community that had always been part of Montefiore, the social experiments as important as anything that happened in the laboratory. He saw a hospital as a place in

which to treat the sick but, also, in which to formulate methods
of improving the public health and to nurture other innovators,
a base from which to seek out those who needed care they could
not afford or find, a platform from which to attack or advise the
political and medical establishments, a school in which to teach
not the usual medical curriculum but a view of medicine and of
society.

He succeeded in his aims through his power of persuasion, his
ability to enlist other people in his projects, his talent as a
salesman of ideas. Barbara Yuncker of the New York *Post* described his modus operandi as "counseling, maneuvering,
placating, prodding, spreading . . . a gift of gab over a baker's
dozen of projects, all aiming at the goal of excellence in medical
care for everyone." Argumentative, stubbornly devoted to a
cause, obsessed with the institution that was the center of his
life, he was rarely still, and never satisfied.

As manager, he always dealt, inside and outside the Hospital,
with independent forces with whom negotiations, conciliation,
bargaining, discussion, and parleying were the only effective
strategies. Even when they were possible, economic threats or
rewards were unlikely to create gentle nursing, diagnostic brilliance, bureaucratic imagination, or philanthropic fervor.
Understanding the difficulties of holding this intricate edifice
together, he was able to persuade the Trustees, government officials, the payers-out of insurance, the faculties of medical
schools, community insurgents, attending physicians, and researchers dedicated to the pursuit of scientific purity to join a
crusade whose aims they did not always grasp or fully approve,
and to give the financial and intellectual support to keep the
enterprise afloat.

Cherkasky successfully rode the waves of a stormy world of
change, creating during his stewardship a different kind of
place. The old Montefiore was not capable of taking advantage
of the new discoveries, the new resources. Under Cherkasky the
tuberculosis sanitarium disappeared, the number of beds in the
buildings on Gun Hill Road actually decreased, while the techniques available for the care of each patient, the number of

highly trained people at each bedside, the machines, the drugs, the lab procedures, multiplied over and over again. The Hospital for Chronic Diseases became the Montefiore Medical Center, an acute-care general hospital, a great teaching institution, which, together with the Albert Einstein College of Medicine, makes up one of the largest and one of the most influential medical complexes in the world.

This careful empire building went along with experiments in the delivery of medicine to an ever-widening circle of social subgroups, to people often forgotten by society and by medicine: prisoners, street-damaged adolescents, the survivors of urban arson and decay. He frequently spoke of the Hospital as a social instrument and did his best to use Montefiore as a base from which to attack social evil, as a platform from which to advise or lecture politicians in City Hall or on Capitol Hill, to bring before them his personal and particular vision of medicine and community.

A man as complex as the medical center he created presided over that lively period when the budget increased sixtyfold, the number of house staff increased by a factor of seventeen, and the number of employees went from 900 to 7,000. The *Daily News* called him "Med Giant Cherkasky . . . long one of the country's most powerful men in medicine." In his years in Montefiore, this physician became both a hero of and a villain to champions of liberal causes in American health care as he goaded a slow-moving giant into becoming a legend of power and wealth and influence, of never-ending change and never-ending social and medical activism.

For all of his professional life he was attacked by the right wing of the medical establishment. His success in building an empire assured attack from the radical left, especially when his vision of utopia differed from current orthodoxy. On a personal level, he aroused, inside and outside the Hospital, loyalty, envy, anger, love, hate, awe, and puzzlement.

Montefiore entered the modern era of medicine with a background of experience and research and with well-trained staff in the very areas that were the central concerns of that era. As

[2 0 3]

infectious diseases succumbed to drugs and vaccines, all hospitals turned their attention to those conditions which had always been the concern of Montefiore—heart disease and cancer. In 1949, Montefiore had 105 beds in its Division of Neoplastic Diseases, more than any other voluntary general hospital in the United States. Almost half of the patients in the Medical Division had diseases of the heart and circulatory system. As did other hospitals, Montefiore was to lose its largest categories of infectious diseases—syphilis and tuberculosis.

The interest in chronic illness remained. Part of the difference was in the way many chronic diseases were treated. Two out of three hospital beds in the country, even those in acute-care institutions, were occupied by people with long-term sickness, most of whom did not remain in the hospital for months or years. They came to the hospital when their problem flared up and then went home to continue life until the next bad episode.

American medicine was going through a period of rapid change in both methods of treatment and methods of financing. More people were entering hospitals for their medical care. In 1940, there were 10 million hospital patients in the country. Ten years later there were 17 million. Part of the increase was the result of the antibiotics that were bringing infection under greater control, part the result of refined surgical techniques, and a considerable portion was the result of wider insurance coverage that allowed more people to pay their hospital bills. In 1940, only 10 million people were covered. By 1950, 87 million people, more than half the population of the United States, had some form of medical insurance. Most of this came as a result of the job-related benefits. Blue Cross was paying out $500 million each year; other insurance companies, $200 million. Combined with government subsidy for building and research, this made health care the country's fourth-largest industry, something like 4 percent of the national income spent on health care.

At the same time the rate of federal subsidy to medical care increased enormously, channeled in ways that benefited the growth of hospitals and medical schools. The Hill-Burton Act provided money for building hospitals; the Veterans Administration continued to expand its facilities. Some government agencies concerned with health, such as the Children's Bureau and the Public Health Service, continued to grow. There was enormous expansion, however, in the most persistent and idiosyncratic aspect of the United States government financing of the health-care establishment: categorical funding based on particular diseases. The National Institutes of Health, each devoted to a particular disease or problem—cancer or heart disease or mental health—flourished, each institute conducting its own programs and backing research projects, usually based in hospitals or medical schools.

American hospitals were entering a period of constant growth, based on fundamental changes in treatment and financial support. Montefiore was caught up in the process. There were characteristics of the old Montefiore: the chronically ill still occupying most of the beds, movies scheduled once a week in the Social Hall, Montefiore still a philanthropic institution, the Trustees dispensing charity in the old ways.

On the other hand, statistics for the ten years from 1944 to 1954 indicate the great changes at the Hospital. Admissions went from 1,725 to 7,119. The average stay on the wards dropped from 160 days to 60; in the private rooms, from 60 days to 13 days. The private and semiprivate service grew enormously, from 468 patients to 4,666. The number of major operations went from 256 to 1,827 and the minor from 674 to 2,551; X-rays from 12,602 to 109,309; outpatient visits from 12,809 to 32,229; lab tests from 21,689 to 170,193. The number of dental visits and procedures tripled because the department was taking care of all the families who were part of the Family Health Maintenance Demonstration. The number of beds had not changed, the budget was about $4 million, of which 84 percent came from private philanthropy or city subsidy. There was a house staff of 66, a "consulting and visiting staff" of 310, 426 nurses, a laboratory staff of 61, and 600 "other employees."

Cherkasky set about changing relationships within the administrative structure of the hospital. To him, the chiefs of divisions were the heart of the matter. Under Bluestone's administration, there had existed a regular joint conference meeting of the chiefs of the divisions and the senior people on the Board of Trustees. Cherkasky did not like that system: "As Chief of Social Medicine I attended those meetings. Often the chiefs had differences among themselves. Each one would present his position to the Board members and press for a decision." He wanted something different: "I gathered the chiefs and I said, 'Look, we are going to constitute a real executive committee, and I'm going to be open with you and honest with you and share with you everything that I know about the hospital and about the Board. I would say to you that we have one of two choices. Either we will sit here and talk through our problems until we agree on a single course of action, and we'll run the Hospital, or we'll continue as we are doing and the Board will run the Hospital.' "

Recruiting gifted chiefs, and supplying them with the resources they required to build their departments, seemed to Cherkasky the central task in creating a first-class general hospital. (A remarkable number of chiefs, when asked why they came to Montefiore, began their answers, "Martin promised . . .") He interested them in coming to his institution by undertaking to fund their research and their special interests. His ability to find resources enabled him to fulfill the promises.

Some of his administrators, appalled by the improvisational nature of the somewhat ramshackle organizational structure he built, dreaming of logic and accountability, accused him of managing his chiefs by bribery. He saw the process as one of meeting their needs as scientists and researchers. In return, he expected only that they would pursue their own and their divisions' interests. He never expected loyalty to his own ends, or even understanding of his goals. He entered each meeting with his chiefs as if it were the first, always anticipating the need for argument and persuasion, always assuming that each chief had uppermost in mind his (or once, in later years, her) own division or departmental concerns. These were the great dukes with whom the king parleyed, not his subjects.

He assumed leadership of an institution in a process of

change. Without any precise blueprints for the future, the imaginative improviser, the opportunist, knew the kind of hospital he wanted to create: "When I became the Director, I was deeply concerned about Montefiore being different from other hospitals in the sense that I wanted it to become something more than the usual first-rate teaching and care institution. I wanted it to be an institution that probed out into the society and which used all of its capabilities to do what I saw its task to be."

The times were not welcoming for social change. Parallel with the great hopes with which the United States entered the postwar era ran a deep streak of fear, a paranoia that threatened to paralyze the nation as a varied series of witch-hunters—Richard Nixon and Joseph McCarthy and the House Un-American Activities Committee—tried to exorcise the demons of Communism that they saw everywhere, generating hysteria that ruined lives and reputations. Montefiore resisted the siege as best it could. Individual physicians assisted colleagues. Places were found on the staff, as they always had been, for people found politically undesirable elsewhere. The Sanitarium provided refuge as a physician called before a congressional committee developed a sudden case of tuberculosis that required prolonged bed rest. Cherkasky found himself the object of visits from the FBI. In later years, he wondered how much of his own activity had been inhibited by the atmosphere of fear. Physicians fleeing the political storms of Europe still found refuge: Edith Kepes, Lucie Adelsberger, Berta Rubinstein.

Cherkasky's basic task in the fifties was to shepherd Montefiore through the change that was already underway from a Hospital for Chronic Diseases to an acute-care hospital. This was a time of revolutionary change in medicine. Antibiotics and vaccines were to conquer huge areas of the territory dominated by infectious diseases and in the process wipe out whole categories of the problems with which Montefiore had been traditionally concerned. Tuberculosis was to be finally contained, syphilis treated with penicillin, rheumatic fever to become a rarity, polio to disappear. Cardiac problems were no longer to be dealt with by bed rest, but by open-heart surgery and pace-makers. This new kind of medicine was much more expensive. He had to find the necessary resources.

Unlike Bluestone, Cherkasky was interested in finances. He liked reading budgets and figuring out how to make the best possible use of available reimbursement, interpreting Blue Cross regulations (still rather loose) so that the category "extraordinary repairs" paid for the remodeling of the interior of a whole building. He saw the capturing and allocation of resources as the essential activity of any administrator, in one stretch of time ridding himself of seven financial officers in seven years until he found someone as quick-witted and creative in the field as himself. He rapidly realized some of the essentials of the hospital business. Like a hotel, a hospital can't make money from empty beds. Heating and lighting an empty ward costs as much as doing the same for a full one. On the other hand, the coming of insurance as the mainstay of hospital financing made thrift a vice, not a virtue. The reimbursement system did not favor an institution that saved money. A hospital was reimbursed for the money it spent. If it cut its per diem costs, the reimbursement was also cut. He also realized that the days of loose regulation on the part of the insurance companies would not last, that he should take advantage of the existing situation. He also knew that he could expand or raise salaries or provide new services if he could persuade the city of New York, which still paid for many days of care for the medically indigent, or Blue Cross to raise payments.

In the fifties, most acute-care hospitals were satisfied if 70 to 80 percent of their beds were filled. For most of its history Montefiore had operated at something like 90 percent capacity, usually with a long waiting list. Cherkasky saw no reason to change. Maximum use of beds meant maximum possibilities for reimbursement and became part of his continuing financial plan, in spite of problems this might create for housekeeping staff or attending physicians waiting for beds for their own patients. He urged doctors to admit patients.

While he encouraged doctors to admit their private patients,

Cherkasky was as opposed as Bluestone to fee-for-service medicine. In 1959 he wrote in *Resident Physician*: ". . . ultimately the complex illnesses we will have to deal with can only be met by pre-paid, comprehensive, preventive-medicine-oriented group practice." Ten years later he declared in an interview: "Fee-for-service is piecework—a professionally undignified way to practice medicine. It's a mechanism of payment almost calculated to seduce the doctor into placing cash before care."

Thus, the modern Montefiore was an institution with a built-in, unresolvable tension between those who saw the physician in private practice as the desirable norm and those who sought different models for the delivery of care. The voluntary attending physicians who brought their patients to the hospital, who did much of the bedside teaching and thought of themselves as the role models for the residents in training, often felt their needs and the needs of their patients were ignored. Medical Board meetings were frequently the scene of complaints about difficulties in obtaining beds for admissions, the forum for complaints that the programs through which the administration reached out to the community created demands for beds and treatment that the hospital could not meet.

Cherkasky managed to walk the tightrope, to keep the centrifugal forces from sending the whole enterprise flying apart, because he was able to bring in the resources, financial and intellectual, that could provide the technology, attract the well-prepared house staff, and support the creative people upon whom both kinds of activities depended.

To replace himself as Chief of the Division of Social Medicine, Cherkasky brought in an old friend from Philadelphia, George Silver, whom Cherkasky had a habit of describing as "the smartest man in the United States." Social medicine is a discipline especially difficult to delineate. Silver decided that at Montefiore social medicine "concerned itself with social factors as they influence medical practice" and meant "principally the concern for problems relating to the organization and administration of medical service." Equally important was the circumstance that the formal Division of Social Medicine at Montefiore, remarkable then and now for standing in equal relationship with the more traditional clinical services, grew not from theory but from programs already in effective existence: "From the standpoint of the Montefiore Hospital, the 'action' qualities of social medicine are paramount, and social medicine is rather like the technology of clinical medicine—the application of clinical medicine to society."

Silver took over the Bluestone-designed Department of Social Medicine to administer social services, Home Care, the Medical Group, the Family Health Maintenance Demonstration, social statistics, and education and research in social medicine and medical care. His background in public health was reflected in the two-year residency program he set up: eight months were spent with the New York City Health Department, eight months at a school of public health, and eight months in administrative training in social medicine.

The Family Health Maintenance Demonstration continued studying the health of two groups of families: the first cared for by a team composed of an internist, a pediatrician, a public health nurse, and a social worker; the control families receiving their care from individual practitioners in the Montefiore Medical Group.

Health is a difficult notion to define. In this case, the researchers decided that health was a capacity to function successfully in four major areas: work, sex, play, and family life. In the end, they found it hard to prove that there was much difference in the health of the two groups. On the other hand, they felt that the "team organization of medical care was successfully demonstrated and seemed highly satisfactory to the patients."

During its period of operation the Demonstration was, according to Silver, "the major national institutional research effort in the field of social medicine" and was the base for teaching social medicine to students at Columbia and later at Einstein, with students and professionals coming from all over the country to study all the department's programs.

One of the oldest Montefiore activities was coming to an end.

When Irving Gottsegen, after a stint at the Columbia School of Public Health and two or three years living in the Green House with the other young administrators at Montefiore, went to Bedford Hills to run the Sanitarium, he found a world still obsessed with fresh air and rest even though the experiments with streptomycin and the other drugs that were to bring the white plague under control were already in progress at Montefiore. About 170 employees cared for 235 patients, divided into two classes: "infirmary," who were in bed at all times, and "ambulant," who were in bed from 9:30 p.m. to 7:15 a.m. and for three rest periods, adding up to five hours, during the day. They were still subject to rules expressed in the manner of schoolteachers: "Plants are the only items allowed on inside windowsills." "The public rooms of the hospital are considered your living room. You would hardly throw paper or bottles on the living room floor in your own home, so please treat our living room in the same way."

The war against card playing continued. This dangerous activity was permissible only between 7:30 p.m. and 9:00 p.m. with "NO card playing allowed at any other time." The struggle against sex was also continued: visiting from floor to floor and building to building was allowed only between patients of the same sex, although the effort to prevent chance encounters while patients strolled the grounds was abandoned. The Occupational Therapy Department taught ceramics, jewelry making, photography, woodworking, and watch and earphone repairing to the ambulant and less strenuous skills to those confined to bed.

The new Chief of the Pulmonary Division, Robert Bloch, had been a close friend and professional colleague of Louis Leiter's since they first met in Chicago in 1927. He had been the first person to actually start work at the new medical school at the University of Chicago, where he worked long and strenuously and against great opposition for the use of X-rays, not only as the primary diagnostic tool in suspected cases of tuberculosis but also as a screening device in seemingly healthy populations —a battle not won until World War II, when the government X-rayed every enlistee and draftee. When he came to Bedford

Hills, Bloch found a Sanitarium still a part of that world of fresh air and discipline and magic ritual, in spite of the chemical revolution. Another anti-tuberculosis drug, isoniazid, appeared, seeming more effective than streptomycin, produced fewer side effects, and could be given by mouth. It could also be given along with streptomycin, a combination more efficient than either drug alone.

As Bloch presided over the careful tests of the new drugs in the green hills of Westchester County, the end result was not clear. During 1953 a series of memos was exchanged among Cherkasky, Silver, and Bloch concerning a "Proposal for a Tuberculosis Home Care Program." Silver was a strong advocate of Home Care. Bloch had doubts, both about Home Care and about the drugs, writing to Silver: "It must be emphasized that our experience now shows that chemotherapy does not shorten the duration of treatment and consequently prolonged treatment may become burdensome, even at home."

The argument went on for three years, with Silver enthusiastically pressing the emotional and practical advantages of the home while Bloch advocated the sanitarium: "While it is true that institutional life holds its disadvantages and irritations, it is equally true that home life threatens with more emotional upheavals. I know that some patients, in fact, find relief in an institution from an unpleasant home situation. This, during the active stage of the disease, is of paramount importance."

The discussion was academic. Cherkasky was intent on building a modern acute-care hospital. For that he needed money. The Sanitarium, built for the poor who could not afford private care, had always cost money. Blue Cross did not cover long-term care. The success of drug therapy was not related to fresh country air or green grass and trees. The Trustees found themselves, for the first time since 1912, involved in large-scale real estate deals. In 1956 the Sanitarium was sold to the Department of Welfare of the City of New York.

The control of tuberculosis affected the doctors as well as the patients. Unlike diabetics, who needed constant, long-term care and supervision from a variety of specialists, tuberculosis patients were cured. Moreover, since new victims could be cured quickly, there would be no further supply of people chronically ill with tuberculosis. The surgeons who had learned their skills operating on tubercular lungs transferred their skills to the growing supply of lungs affected by cancer. There was no longer a need for the large numbers of physicians who had specialized in tuberculosis.

In the Bronx, the fifties were an era of expansion of facilities and services. The children of Montefiore were finally recognized as a separate medical entity with the invitation to Dr. Milton Grand to return. As a resident in the thirties, he had disliked the unbending rigidities of Bluestone's administration. In 1953 Grand came back to the Bronx, and established the first Pediatric Service at Montefiore, with forty beds in the Rosenthal Pavilion, which was under construction.

By the end of 1954, there were plans for another division that had never previously existed at Montefiore, although many patients had always needed—and sometimes received—this kind of care. Psychiatry was to be housed in the new Klau Pavilion, with facilities for outpatients and twenty-two inpatient beds. This was probably the most carefully planned of the new services and a division which closely followed the original blueprints over a remarkable length of time. A committee of Board members, physicians, and "two distinguished members of the community," Ralph and David Straus, spent two years considering the kind of service appropriate to deal with what was by then the leading cause of hospitalization in the country. The group decided that "to round out Montefiore's program in the field of patient care, education and research, it was essential that an adequate psychiatric division be created to take its place alongside medicine, surgery and other divisions as a major hospital activity."

This would be an essential service to patients already in the Hospital: ". . . in meeting the problems of the chronically sick which is our major responsibility we have long recognized that this kind of illness not only threatens the individual's physical being but also threatens his emotional and family life; so that one of the responsibilities of the Division of Psychiatry will be to work with physicians in every area of the Hospital and in every division of the Hospital to enable the best psychiatric care to be integrated with the best in organic medicine to meet the total needs of the patient.

"We also hope to make a psychiatric orientation and a basic understanding of the role of psychiatry in the practice of medicine a part of the training program for every resident in the Hospital no matter what service he may be on."

The first Chief was Dr. Seymour Perlin, who had served at the National Institute of Health as Chief of the Psychosomatic Service and as Chief of the Section on Psychiatry of the Clinical Science Laboratory. A Psychosomatic Service had already been set up as an integral part of the Department of Medicine, under the direction of Dr. Hyman Bakst, an internist, and Dr. Janet Kennedy, a psychoanalyst. Each month a different resident was assigned to the service and given the task of doing a thorough medical work-up on an entering patient, with special attention paid to the emotional factors that cause or affect disease. Twice a week the resident presented the findings at a staff seminar attended by a social worker, the nurse in charge of the ward, and other physicians. Then the patient was interviewed by Dr. Kennedy, the purpose "to reveal and demonstrate how the unconscious factors in a patient's personality can cause or contribute to illness," followed by a discussion of the interaction of the medical and psychological forces bearing on the patient's problems. The conferences became a regular part of the training of residents in medicine.

The School of Practical Nursing continued to flourish, and to be a source of training and employment for black men and women. In 1952, Carl Owens of Brooklyn, a twenty-seven-year-old former textile printer and one of the eleven men in a class of seventy-five, received the Board of Trustees award as the outstanding student. In 1956, ninety-two women and nine men made up the largest class ever. The age range was wide, from seventeen to fifty, with most over twenty-five. The low cost (students paid only a $15 fee for books and received a small living allowance) and low educational requirements (the equivalent of an elementary school education was the minimum) enabled many who would not have been eligible for any other kind of training to enter the program.

At the same time, great efforts were made to attract registered nurses. The country was going through one of its recurrent nursing shortages. To attract a full complement of nurses, Montefiore opened a Day Care Center for their children, and with the help of the Bloomingdale family, who had served on the Board of Trustees for generations, built housing for nurses—not the single rooms of other days, but studio apartments.

Nursing was never to lose the need for the simple, caring skills: the need for hands that fed and washed and touched. Other developments in the Hospital called for a constantly increasing level of scientific knowledge and ability to deal with crisis medicine. Those new operating rooms were to require O.R. nurses of formidable skills.

Montefiore was now an institution well supplied with operating rooms, with a brilliant new Chief of Surgery (Elliott Hurwitt), and a history of performing much less surgery than other hospitals the same size. In the Hospital for Chronic Diseases, surgery was more an adjunct to the other services than an independent activity and was usually performed by a visitor from Mount Sinai. In the modern era, surgery was to remain a close working partner of the other disciplines. With patients being admitted from the Medical Group, the number of procedures was bound to increase. The fifties, however, were to bring spectacular developments in surgery out of one of the traditionally important medical services: cardiology.

Under Louis Leiter as Chief of Medicine, research activities were developing the tools that would enable Montefiore to join the coming revolution in heart surgery. Under his direct supervision as a kidney expert, research in diuretics and kidney function continued to bring improvements in the management of cardiac patients, while Dr. Doris Escher worked to improve an essential technique in the modern diagnosis and treatment of the heart: cardiac catheterization, the threading of a tube through an artery or vein into the vessels and chambers of the heart so that the pressure and flow of blood could be accurately measured. The physician could also use the catheter for the injection of radiopaque substances that would show up on an angiographic X-ray. When Escher first came to Montefiore in 1942, cardiac catheterization was in its infancy. By 1946, under Louis Leiter she and Raymond Weston were running a research program which by 1950 had become the second or third cath lab in the city and the first to use the technique on young babies and newborns, ready to become the essential backup to cardiac surgery.

The study of the heart and the pathways of the blood was a group activity at Montefiore, and often highly competitive. Dr. Henry Haimovici, who became a world-renowned expert on vascular surgery, thirty-five years later was still brooding over his suspicion that Adrian Kantrowitz (later a world-renowned heart surgeon), as a resident at Montefiore, had stolen a batch of the cats on which Haimovici planned to operate. Kantrowitz devised a model of an artificial heart apparatus. Antol Herskowitz, the hospital photographer, made a movie of it in action.

In the early fifties experimental heart surgery on humans was a reality in several centers in the United States for conditions such as mitral stenosis, the constriction or narrowing of the mitral valve of the heart. Hurwitt maintained that "in no other field of surgery is the group concept so important." At Montefiore, any case being considered for cardiovascular surgery was reviewed by the Cardiovascular Group, composed of internists, cardiologists, cardiovascular physiologists, anesthesiologists, pathologists, and radiologists. Each case was also formally presented to the regularly scheduled cardiovascular conferences, where differences of opinion were "freely aired and sometimes warmly contested."

By the end of 1952 Hurwitt was able to report that thirty patients had been operated on at Montefiore for mitral stenosis. Only two had died.

Teamwork was essential in the operating room. Hurwitt described it: "A cardiologist is in constant attendance, monitoring the electrocardiogram and quickly picking up and correcting any changes. Continuous oximetry is an aid both to the anesthesiologist and to the electrocardiographer. Apparatus for taking pressure measurements directly from the heart during operation and for electrical defibrillation (stabilizing the heartbeat) further adds to the assembly. One member of the house staff is assigned solely to measuring blood loss and supervising the fluid and transfusion apparatus."

This was ultimately blind surgery. The heart continued beating and the blood flowing and it was the finger of the surgeon that finally entered the valve and pushed at the obstruction. Hurwitt reported that "in no case in our series so far has it been necessary to use a knife to effect opening of the valve, although such instruments are always available." The operation was palliative, not a cure. The valve was not replaced, but most patients found their health and the quality of their lives vastly improved.

For early heart surgery speed had again become one of the surgeon's most important skills. Hypothermia was used: lowering the patient's temperature by immersion in ice water, slowing the body's functions enough to give the surgeon about six minutes in which to work. The answer to the time dilemma was to be the heart-lung machine, which took over the task of pumping and oxygenating the body's blood supply while the heart was actually stopped by chemical injection and the surgeon could work by sight instead of feel. In the fifties many centers in the United States and Europe were busy developing their own versions of the machines. The Montefiore group under the leadership of Dr. George Robinson built their own pump oxygenator, a complicated series of gears and tubes which carried off blood before it reached the heart, purified it with oxygen as the lungs do, and sent it back to circulate in the arteries. The heart-lung machine was used in a series of operations to correct congenital heart defects in children. The risks involved in stopping the heart were enormous, and as the length of time that the patient remained unconscious increased, the role of the anesthetist became more and more complicated. Indeed, the whole process would have been impossible without the increasingly sophisticated techniques used by the Anesthesiology Service under Dr. Edith Kepes. As the surgeons worked, the anesthetist checked the level of unconsciousness, the oxygen level of the blood, the hemoglobin level, the blood level, kidney function, and other signals from a body undergoing severe stress.

Ever since the beginning of the industrial revolution, social reformers have been concerned that machines would replace people. The replacement has not occurred in medicine. The more machines that came into the hospital, the more people were required to tend the machines and the patients. The machines that came into the operating room brought crowds of people with them.

The difficulties of hospital planning were well illustrated by the construction of the operating rooms. Bluestone and the Board had guessed well when they assumed that the number of surgical procedures would increase. They had planned, however, in the late forties, for much less complicated surgery than quickly became the reality. Almost from the time the new operating rooms opened, there were complaints about over-crowding, not so much because there were not enough rooms as because they were too small to comfortably accommodate the machines and the people now a necessary part of the team. As the length of time needed for each procedure increased, operating room time became harder to allocate. After these difficult procedures, patients were kept under observation in the recovery room, which also became overcrowded. The operating suite was outdated almost from the time it opened. Complaints about the situation from surgeons, especially the attending staff, quickly became a fixture of Medical Staff meetings.

Hurwitt was Chief during a period when surgery went from being a minor part of life at Montefiore to an activity that took a large part of the time and resources of the Hospital and quickly became surgery on the frontiers of science. By 1959 the team (now eighteen at each procedure) was performing two open-heart operations each week. On the other hand, surgical residents were sent elsewhere to observe tonsillectomies and deliveries.

In the meantime, another invention had become available to the heart surgeons. One of the people who worked on the heart-lung machine was Dr. Seymour Furman, who graduated from Downstate Medical School in 1955 to begin an internship at Montefiore. Working half-time in the cardiac catheterization laboratory, he learned cardiac cath techniques, measuring intracardiac pressures and cardiac output. His first task in the open-heart surgery program was to help build the bubble oxygenator.

The great danger in heart surgery was, of course, that the heart would accidentally stop either during or after surgery, and various forms of electrical stimulus had been developed at the University of Minnesota and other centers to restart the heart. Furman was given several dogs on which to duplicate these methods of cardiac pacing. His own limited training in electronics, acquired building radios as a boy, convinced him that the wire he planned to insert should be insulated. He threaded the stainless-steel wire through polyethylene tubing. The other essential was to reduce the output voltage to a safe level. With help from a commercial firm, Furman built a voltage reducer that effectively stepped output down to a tenth.

Furman felt that "the technique of stimulating the heart directly with the myocardial wires and the external stimulator clearly was ready to work in the operating and recovery rooms and the work seemed to be ended." Hurwitt suggested to him that funds were available and that he might want to try other projects with the hardware, the recording devices, the animal lab technicians, and the dogs that were left.

He proceeded to stop the beating of dogs' hearts and to restart them with electric shocks to the heart muscle. His experience in cardiac cath suggested that he could lead the wires through the veins to the heart. His polyethylene tubing became a cardiac catheter, inserted through the dogs' jugular veins, taking a braided copper wire through to the hearts. For about three months Furman repeated his experiments with his dogs, proving over and over again that pacing through the veins worked, without exciting any particular interest in the research laboratories. Finally, in the spring of 1958, he told the story to John B. Schwedel, the Chief of Cardiology. According to Furman: "Dr. Schwedel grasped the importance of the technique instantly, became extremely excited, and assured me that clinical trial was mandatory and that he would help me. He spoke to the Chief of Surgery and told him that the technique was not only of potentially immense value but a thrilling possibility and that the two of them, the Chief of Surgery and the Chief of Cardiology, should take the responsibility of fostering the development. He began to look for a suitable patient."

A difficulty with medical experiments is that they usually have to be carried out on extremely sick patients. The first patient was sixty-nine years old, had already had complete heart block for eleven years, and was in the hospital with cancer of the colon. Furman's pacemaker was used successfully to keep the man's heart beating during the operation in which his colon was resectioned. Pacing was stopped after the surgery. The patient died after a second operation during which the pacemaker was not used.

The next subject was a seventy-six-year-old man who had been in chronic congestive heart failure for many years following rheumatic heart disease. The electrode catheter was threaded through a vein in his left arm to his heart; a second electrode, a stainless-steel suture, was embedded under the skin of his chest. The pacemaker proceeded to stimulate his heart and he was returned to his room. Two months later he could get out of bed. The pacemaker was the size of a large radio. It was placed on a wheeled table, a fifty-foot cord attached, and the patient, with a nurse at his side, walked the corridor pushing his pacemaker ahead of him. Thirteen weeks and five days after it had been inserted, the catheter was withdrawn, the heart beating regularly without stimulation. He returned home, the first patient anywhere to leave a hospital after transvenous pacing, to live for two and a half more years. During the next eighteen months, seventeen patients underwent transvenous pacing, two of them ultimately living for more than nineteen years and one for more than twenty.

A year later the pacemaker was transistorized. The patient carried this model, weighing about two pounds and powered by three mercury batteries, around in his hand. In December 1961, the size was down to that of a cigarette pack and the device was implanted under the patient's skin for the first time. By 1966, about 160 patients had been treated at Montefiore with cardiac pacemakers.

Under Hurwitt's leadership, other forms of surgery flourished. In 1958, Dr. Henry Heimlich (later to achieve fame as the inventor of the Heimlich Maneuver for use with people choking on food) devised a procedure to help patients suffering from cancer of the esophagus and unable to eat. A long narrow strip was cut from the wall of the stomach, with the point of attachment serving as a hinge on which the tube swung up toward the throat. Once the tube was in place and connected at the neck the patient was able to eat again. In a second operation the cancerous esophagus was removed, offering hope of actual cure. The same operation was used to help a woman who had not been able to swallow for twenty-nine years after accidentally drinking lye. For all that time she had been fed through a tube directly into her stomach. After the surgery she was able to swallow normally.

In 1958, Michael Lewin, head of the Plastic Surgery Service, was asked to perform a cleft palate operation on an inmate at Sing Sing Prison. This led to a continuing program, with sixty procedures performed in two years by Lewin and a team that included Dr. Eugene Gottlieb and a resident, Dr. Ravello Argamaso. Once a week they went up to the prison hospital and operated on a series of congenital defects and disfiguring scars, the aim being to assist in the rehabilitation of prisoners. Lewin pointed out that "plastic surgery is not a cure-all, but we are convinced, from the successes we already have had, that it can be of great benefit to seriously handicapped or abnormal-looking individuals."

In 1960, there arrived the device that was to become a feature of television hospital dramas, the cardiac cart. Medical and surgical residents were appointed on a monthly rotation to staff the cart, which was equipped with an electronic pacemaker, a defibrillator, an electrocardiograph, and an oxygen supply. The first time that a nurse reported to the switchboard that a patient's heart had stopped, Drs. Martin Goldman and Itamar Salamon responded. The former gave mouth-to-mouth resuscitation while the other opened the chest and massaged the heart. Drs. Harry Gross and Ira Rubin arrived with the cart, and Dr. Frank Davidson inserted the pacemaker. The patient was discharged four weeks later.

American medicine was firmly set on a path toward specialization, and that was reflected in changes in the structure of Montefiore. Perry B. Hudson came from Columbia (where he retained his post as professor of zoology) to head the Urology Service, now one of the ten services in the Division of Surgery. The Division of Medicine included the Cardiology, Dermatology, and Gastroenterology Services. There were now thirteen divisions: Anesthesiology, Diagnostic, Radiology, Laboratories, Medicine, Neoplastic Medicine, Neurology, Neurosurgery, Pediatrics, Psychiatry, Pulmonary Medicine, Rehabilitation Medicine, Social Medicine, and Surgery as well as three departments: Dental Surgery, Hematology, and Radiotherapy.

In 1960, research grants reached a record high with almost two hundred projects all told, with funding from the United States Health Service ($575,000), the Atomic Energy Commission, the National Heart Association, the National Multiple Sclerosis Society, the Rockefeller Foundation, and the city of New York.

Studies in metabolism were under the general direction of Louis Leiter, who with Dr. Jack Grossman was studying the metabolism of potassium and the influence of hormones on dietary metabolism. Herta Spencer, Laszlo's widow, headed a team investigating the metabolism of calcium and strontium 90, a by-product of the testing of atomic bombs. Harry Zimmerman was researching the effect on the brain of an inadequate oxygen supply and, using the electron microscope, the link between blood vessels and brain function. He achieved an international reputation for his contributions in neuropathology in such areas as the neurologic effects of vitamin deficiency, chemically induced gliomas, and multiple sclerosis. He attracted students from all over the world, who later returned to their own countries to head an extraordinary number of major diagnostic and research laboratories and academic departments.

The Trustees, while adjusting to this new Hospital, where they could no longer decide admissions or discharges, continued old interests. Philanthropy was still an important source of funds. The Radiotherapy Department under Charles Botstein and Diagnostic Radiology under Harold Jacobson were particularly dependent on technology and the novel and expensive equipment constantly under development. Mrs. Belle Binswanger, who had spent so much time with the children in the twenties and thirties and was now over ninety, gave $30,000 to buy a machine which developed and delivered dry X-ray films in six minutes, ready for interpretation by a radiologist. Henry Moses gave $150,000 to pay for a six-ton, 35-million-volt betatron named Asklepitron, after the ancient Greek healer. The machine fired high-speed electrons at cancer cells. Dr. Botstein explained the advantages over X-rays. "Even at high power, electrons can be controlled in a more precise manner than X-rays. The depth of penetration of the beam is determined by the speed of the emitted electrons and the path the beam takes through the body can be concentrated by placing magnets along its path. In this way, healthy tissues behind the diseased part and surrounding the path are spared from damage."

Dr. Jacob Spira, a physicist in the Radiotherapy Department, spent two months in Switzerland studying the machine, which was then sent from Baden to Rotterdam by train, to New York by ship, to the Bronx by truck, and finally, with the help of a 100-foot crane, lowered through a hole in the Montefiore roof and installed behind seven-foot-thick concrete walls.

Another Board member, with strong family connections to Montefiore, brought scientific knowledge to Board deliberations. The grandson of the first President of the Auxiliary, the son of Fred Stein, William Stein was a distinguished scientist who ultimately won a Nobel Prize in chemistry for his work at the Rockefeller Institute.

In the years when Cherkasky was taking charge of Montefiore, many people on the staff were devoting a major part of their efforts to the creation of the first Jewish medical school in the United States, with Samuel Belkin, President of Yeshiva University, its godfather. The idea of a medical school was attractive to him as a device for adding both prestige and money to his institution, beset, as it was, by chronic financial troubles. To many physicians and scientists whose careers had been distorted by prejudice, a Jewish medical school was an old dream. They now had a prosperous Jewish community whose origin was Eastern European and who had never believed, as many in the German Jewish community had believed, that assimilation was a possible solution. They were prepared to build totally Jewish institutions instead of attempting to infiltrate the gentile schools. Not everybody was enthusiastic. Louis Leiter opposed the idea of a Jewish school.

By 1951 Yeshiva University received a charter to establish a medical school from the state of New York. Harry Zimmerman took a two-year leave of absence to become acting dean of the new school. The question of a name for the school came up. Someone suggested the name of Joseph Goldberger, to honor the American Jewish physician who had found the cause of pellagra. A small group traveled to Princeton to ask Albert Einstein for permission to use his name. Professor Einstein demurred, on the grounds that he was not a physician. Goldberger was mentioned as an alternative. Einstein looked puzzled. "Who is Goldberger?" he asked, thus proving the value of his own easily recognized and glamorous name.

Marcus Kogel, who became the first Dean of Albert Einstein College of Medicine, played a decisive part in founding, locating, and shaping the school. As Commissioner of Hospitals of the City of New York, he had presided over the building of the Bronx Municipal Hospital in the northeast Bronx, and the designers of the college were able to buy land next to the hospital on which to build their school. Public officials cooperated, even agreeing to the exchange of a block of land on Staten Island for a parcel of city-owned land in the Bronx to complete the package. The building of the school and its use of the city hospital (and the patients there) for teaching and training students was seen as a way of upgrading a city hospital and bringing better medical care to the people of the Bronx. The college opened in 1955 with fifty-six students.

As Dean, Kogel was determined that this fledgling should become, as quickly as possible, one of the top-ranking medical schools in the United States. He also recognized that prestige and money went to the schools involved in basic research. The federal government, through the National Institutes of Health, was now giving large-scale grants for medical school-based research, and in these heady postwar years of faith in science as the answer to humanity's ills, the laboratory scientist was revered. Kogel's policy worked. The college quickly rose to the first rank and for many years received more federal money than any other medical school.

The Albert Einstein College of Medicine was set on a course of competing, not by being different, but by doing supremely well those things already being done at medical schools, with, from the beginning, a philosophy at variance with Montefiore's traditional concern for family and society and with Cherkasky's efforts to change the way in which medicine was delivered.

Meanwhile, the Jewish hospitals of New York City continued along their divergent pathway. Most of the great teaching hospitals in the country were associated with university medical schools. The Jewish hospitals became "teaching hospitals" because they were not associated with medical schools. The best physicians, whether salaried or voluntary, were often at those hospitals because they were not acceptable at academic centers; the interns and residents were there because they could not find openings at other hospitals. The large Jewish hospitals fostered teaching programs out of self-defense.

In the late fifties less than 60 percent of the patients in Federation hospitals in New York City were Jewish, most of them paying their own way, out of their pockets or through insurance.

They made up only about one quarter of all the Jewish hospital patients in the city. On the other hand, of the 219 interns in the nine Federation hospitals, all but 21 were Jewish. Seventy percent of the 524 residents were Jewish. The raison d'être of Jewish hospitals as training and career centers for Jewish professionals was clear.

The training programs were of high quality. Federation hospitals, with the assistance of Federation subsidy and encouragement, had followed Montefiore's lead in establishing full-time clinical chiefships. There were now twenty-nine of them in eight of the Federation hospitals. Montefiore led the way with nine, followed by Mount Sinai with six. Federation hospitals had attracted about 84 percent of the interns they had chosen through the National Intern Matching Program. About half of these interns were in the upper or middle third of their classes. Eighty percent of the best-qualified interns went to Mount Sinai or Montefiore. Half of the Federation residents were at the same two hospitals, which together absorbed 70 percent of the $2.5 million spent for research and teaching fellowships in Federation hospitals.

On the other hand, there were signs pointing to fundamental changes. Jewish physicians were finding that internships, residencies, and staff appointments were opening up to them in non-Jewish hospitals, partly the result of the development of a more open society, partly because many hospitals in the immediate postwar years had established or expanded training programs to meet the influx of returning veterans and did not wish to shrink their size now that the demand was over.

The teaching programs at Montefiore were expanding at a time when many hospitals were having trouble filling their internship and residency slots. To meet the postwar need for training, hospitals had created programs and now the United States had twice as many medical internships as there were students graduating. Medical schools had not expanded and students found themselves under pressures and enticements to accept appointments. To sort out the resulting confusion, the Association of American Medical Colleges, the American Medical Association, and the American Hospital Association set up a centralized system, the National Matching Program, to which all graduates applied.

By 1959, 128 residents and fellows and 32 interns were in training at Montefiore. Approved residencies existed in anesthesiology, medicine, neoplastic diseases, neurology, neurosurgery, ophthalmology, pathology, pulmonary diseases, physical medicine and rehabilitation, radiology, radiotherapy, social medicine, surgery, and thoracic surgery. While the only residency carried on in collaboration with Albert Einstein was neurosurgery, there was constant cross-fertilization of talent. Charles Botstein came from Albert Einstein to become head of the Department of Radiotherapy, joining Harold Jacobson, Chief of Radiology.

Cherkasky followed both Jewish hospital tradition and the Montefiore tradition in building up his teaching programs. He had another purpose. He knew that his brand of social medicine, his opposition to fee-for-service, his desire to extend medical care to all those cut off by financial and social circumstance, ran counter to the mainstream of medicine, Jewish or gentile. He could only impress an audience if he spoke from the security of a hospital thoroughly respected in the scientific community. He could protect and fund his favorite programs, Social Medicine, Home Care, the Medical Group, and the others that were to follow if he was seen as running a highly successful institution, and he could teach his point of view only in a teaching hospital.

Thus, in the 1950s Montefiore expanded rapidly, not in the number of beds, but in the services offered to patients and the teaching programs which attracted residents and faculty. Buildings went up quickly: the Rosenthal Pavilion and then the Klau Pavilion, service buildings, housing for staff. The surrounding community became accustomed, although not happily, to the distinctive marks of the Cherkasky reign: noise and dust and the sounds of buildings either in the process of demolition or rising rapidly where once were green grass and flowers. One of the aims of construction was achieved: the elimination of the long wards. All the patients were ultimately cared for in one-, two-, or four-bed rooms, with no distinction between paying and non-paying patients.

More money was coming to hospitals than ever before. Little of it, however, trickled down to the people who scrubbed the floors and washed the dishes and made the beds. Salaries were so low that many fully employed hospital workers were eligible for welfare. The starting wage for porters and maids in voluntary hospitals was $35 a week, $20 less than in municipal hospitals, which were more amenable to political pressure.

Leon Davis, of the Retail Drug Employees Local 1199 of the Retail, Wholesale and Department Store Union, decided that something had to be done about these most exploited of workers. This "powerful, passionate man" as Cherkasky described him, driven by an anger on behalf of all the oppressed of the world, a son of Russian Jewish radicalism, set out to improve the condition of a group of people at the bottom of the economic ladder, many of them female, many black or Hispanic, recent immigrants from the poverty belts of the United States, the South, or Puerto Rico, the least skilled, the least experienced in formal organization. In so doing, Davis was attempting to organize a whole industry that had never been touched before. He needed a breakthrough in a major institution.

Montefiore had a reputation for progressive social thinking. Cherkasky was known as a thorn in the side of organized medicine. The Board of Trustees, on the other hand, was a group of conservative businessmen and bankers. They were not accustomed to thinking favorably of unions and they were now in a position to resist a union, secure in the support of the community, their peers on other hospital boards, and the full sanction of the law. The Chairman of the Board, Victor Riesenfeld, had been one of the major negotiators in the textile industry. The most bitter opposition, however, came from other hospitals.

Unsuccessful attempts had been made to organize Montefiore in the late forties and early fifties. Davis' drive succeeded partly because his people understood the peculiar structure of the

Hospital. They organized department by department: nutrition, nurse's aides, and so on, concentrating on the blue-collar and service workers, the organizers as ethnically varied as their targets.

Beginning in December 1957, 1199 mounted a full-scale attack, opening up a headquarters across the street, signing up members, pulling lunchtime demonstrations. By the following August, out of 900 workers, 500 had signed union cards. (Registered nurses and physicians were not counted as workers.)

Montefiore was operating at a deficit of $1.3 million. The deficit would double if the hospital paid wages comparable to those in industry. If wages were to be increased and guaranteed by a union contract, money had to be found. Montefiore's peculiar financial history suggested the solution. During most of the institution's existence, paying patients had never provided a large portion of income. The city of New York had always provided a subsidy for indigent patients, and administrators were accustomed to bargaining over the amount of that subsidy. Cherkasky suggested an increase in the subsidy to pay for the increased wages demanded by the union. Mayor Robert Wagner was sympathetic to unions, but for him to thus sanction and underwrite the existence of this upstart in a field so long regarded as sacrosanct, some kind of public pressure was necessary. The Board of Trustees was also not likely to yield easily, especially as their peers on other hospital boards brought pressure to bear to maintain a united anti-union front. Davis set about creating a wave of public sympathy. In the wake of *Brown* v. *Topeka*, the civil rights movement was gaining momentum, and black politicians and ministers and the *Amsterdam News* took up the 1199 banner. *El Diario* rallied the Spanish-speaking. Mo Foner, Davis' second-in-command, enlisted New York *Post* columnist James Wechsler and appealed to the New York *Times*. The union asked for support from Eleanor Roosevelt and Senator Herbert H. Lehman. Roosevelt used her column, "My Day," to comment on the hardships of hospital workers, and both of them wrote friendly personal letters to Riesenfeld asking him to look into the problem. Harry Van

Arsdale, President of New York City's Central Labor Council, came out in strong support and helped pressure Wagner to make a financial settlement.

Cherkasky himself had doubts about exactly how the management of the Hospital was to be shared with the union, what aspects of working conditions were appropriate subjects for the bargaining table, whether patients' lives would be put at risk. In late November, Davis wrote him a letter which overcame his lingering uncertainties. Davis admitted that Montefiore was the union's one great hope, that total resistance could destroy the union and "defeat these workers [and] destroy their hopes for better conditions now and in the future."

In early December 1958 the union met and threatened a strike. Riesenfeld and Van Arsdale asked the mayor to intervene. He called an emergency meeting, and with the city agreeing privately to raise the subsidy for ward patients from $16 to $20 a day, Montefiore agreed to recognize 1199 as "the sole collective bargaining agent pending a certification election . . . and agreement dealing with all issues." On December 30, when an election was held, two thirds of the 900 workers eligible to vote chose 1199 and three months later the first contract was signed.

Before another year was over, there was a forty-six-day strike at seven voluntary hospitals. Five years later, the union won collective bargaining rights under New York State's Labor Relations Act. Cherkasky's assessment was that "Leon Davis has done something spectacular for a group of disenfranchised people, a very large group, because he has obviously affected not only those places which are unionized, but those places which are not. Everybody's handling of workers and pay and everything else is just infinitely better."

The health-care industry became a source not just of jobs for blacks and Hispanics and other minority groups but of jobs with security, benefits, and the possibility of training and advancement. To Cherkasky, the improvement in wages and working conditions that the union contract brought led also to an improvement in community health. His Depression-sharpened consciousness always saw decent jobs as more necessary to health than any amount of medical care.

The settlement also fitted his view of the financial future of hospitals, the money for support to come more and more from government and less and less from philanthropy or out of the pockets of patients.

CHAPTER
16
Urbi et Orbi

Cherkasky entered the sixties exuberantly, busy nurturing the growth of his own institution and doing his best to improve the delivery of health care in general, constantly flying back and forth to Washington seeking funds for Montefiore or testifying before congressional committees on medical matters, his advice frequently sought by state, local, and federal officials. When it was unsought he had no hesitancy in expressing his opinion.

Trying to rally others to his cause, he addressed an American Public Health Association meeting urging action: "The timidity with which Public Health people approach medical care does justice to their recognition of the violent conflict ahead, but does not either meet the need or reflect the courage and boldness which were the hallmarks of Public Health."

Convinced that public health people had a point of view about medical care that involved a concern for the common good, while most hospital administrators received a training that was purely technical and saw their mission as that of serving the desires of physicians or boards, he appealed to his audience to become more than advice givers, to become hospital administrators.

He developed a close working relationship with a man who followed that path. Ray Trussell spent a career alternating as a teacher in the Columbia School of Public Health, as a hospital administrator, and as Hospitals Commissioner of the City of New York. The pair collaborated on many an effort to improve medical care for the poor of New York City.

In the late fifties, Cherkasky described what he saw during half a year as an unpaid consultant to Trussell: ". . . the hospital [the old Lincoln in the South Bronx] had only two electrocardiograph machines, one of them broken, to serve 400 inpatients and more than 1,000 outpatients each day. At another city hospital, Morrisania, intravenous infusions for critically ill patients had to be cut off for 12 hours each night because there was no one to keep an eye on them."

Most cities in the United States had, at most, one public hospital. Many cities paid voluntary hospitals to take care of their indigent in "charity wards." New York was a city readier to take care of its poor than most regions in the country, ready to spend money on health and education, to build city hospitals and city colleges, public schools and public clinics and public housing.

In 1960 there were 150 voluntary, municipal, and proprietary hospitals in New York City, not counting state and federal institutions or nursing homes. Between them, the municipal and voluntary hospitals had about 50,000 beds, in which they took care of a million patients each year. There were about 7.5 million visits each year to the clinics and emergency rooms. There were now twenty-two municipal hospitals with 18,000 beds run by the Department of Hospitals under a commissioner, most of the buildings shabby, dirty, and outdated, lacking basic equipment and poorly staffed. In the Bronx, 40 percent of the hospital beds were in municipal institutions, the highest proportion in any borough. Twenty-five percent of the population of the Bronx was black and Hispanic, many poor and dependent on city hospitals for care.

Morrisania, built as the Bronx General Hospital in 1929, with an early history of excellence, shared in the general decline of city hospital quality after World War II when young physicians coming back for residency training turned away from city hospitals, looking for places in institutions that were part of or affiliated with universities. At the same time, an influx of graduates of foreign medical schools entered the United States looking for training. Many, whether because of inferior training, language problems, or prejudice, could not meet the competition at the better voluntary hospitals and drifted to the city hospitals.

The increasing number of people covered by health insurance avoided the wards of city hospitals and sought the private and semiprivate rooms of voluntary hospitals. In turn, they were followed by physicians who preferred to spend their time visiting their patients and donating their teaching service efforts to ward patients in the same hospitals, less and less willing to teach in city hospitals that lacked equipment, were dirty and crowded, and where communication with patients was hampered by language barriers. Specialists such as radiologists and pathologists spent fewer hours at the deteriorating facilities. Elderly visiting physicians who died or retired were not replaced. Thus, as the house staff needed more and more supervision, they received less and less.

The National Intern Matching Program arrived, and the least desirable hospitals, a status that New York City hospitals were fast approaching, had less and less hope of filling their places. Montefiore, in spite of its lack of a strong medical school affiliation (by now the connection with Columbia was almost nonexistent in practice), never had problems filling internships and residencies. Its reputation, built up over many years, of investing time and money in research and teaching, by a staff of full-time salaried physicians, ensured that it always "made its match," filling slots with the most desirable candidates.

The relative attractiveness of Morrisania and Montefiore as places to train was indicated by their ability to attract interns. From 1955 to 1962, Montefiore filled all its slots. Morrisania found two "matches" in 1956, and none in any of the other years.

The inadequacy of care at Morrisania was indicated in a history taken by a resident who shared the patient's inability to deal with the English language: An eighty-four-year-old white male patient was seen in the emergency room on March 6, 1960. In the space provided for a brief history was written "7 East" (one of the four medical wards). The admitting diagnosis was "medical observation". The next note on the patient's chart was by the ward resident: ". . . we don't know how old is the patient but looks very old, and was admitted from the E.R. with the usually diagnosis of medical observation . . . no history could be taken because the patient does not speak english and no relative are over here."

As usual, the city hospitals were the frequent subjects of studies, and two of those published in 1960 recommended affiliation between city and voluntary hospitals as a means of upgrading the level of intern and residency training and the quality of patient care. Ray Trussell (as Commissioner of Hospitals) asked Montefiore to become involved.

Cherkasky attempted to upgrade the level of care at Morrisania the first year with a modest program involving one surgical resident. The next year, six residents participated, and the next, fifteen, while members of Montefiore's attending staff were assigned to key teaching positions. As of July 1, 1962, Montefiore assumed contractual responsibility for full-time direction of all medical services and for training house staff.

One result of Montefiore's involvement at Morrisania was that the vague admitting diagnosis of "medical observation" became less common, going from thirty-five in 1960 to eleven in 1961. Another result was that the number of X-rays went up. In 1960, 61 percent of all patients admitted with heart disease did not have a diagnostic chest film; in 1961, this figure was only 38 percent. In 1960, 28 percent of patients admitted with respiratory problems did not have X-rays taken; in 1961 this was only 5 percent. Lab tests showed significant increases between the two dates. The length of time that patients stayed in the hospital increased, and the number of progress notes on the charts doubled. Pelvic and rectal exams showed no increase: one resident explained that he couldn't do a rectal exam because there were no rubber gloves on the floor and none to be found anywhere else in spite of repeated requests, and another did not do a pelvic exam on a female patient because he could not get a nurse as chaperone, necessary under hospital rules.

In true Montefiore tradition, the number of autopsies went up from 21 percent to 41 percent. Also in the Montefiore tradition was the increase in referral of patients for follow-up care to the outpatient clinics, Home Care, nursing homes, or other hospitals, from 24 percent to 43 percent.

In 1960, the six residents whose notes appeared most often on charts on the medical wards came from the Dominican Republic, Germany, Cuba, the Philippines, and Turkey. The six whose notes appeared most often the following year came from medical schools in the New York area. Full-time directors of service were appointed: Drs. Samuel Standard (Surgery), Abraham Tamis (Ob/Gyn), David Grayzel (Pathology and Laboratories), Max Schapira (Anesthesiology), and Wilhelm Zeev Stern (Diagnostic Radiology).

Morrisania had trouble attracting nurses as well as physicians. When Bob Bloom went there as an administrator in 1965, there were 400 beds and 87 registered nurses. The city was not paying salaries comparable with those in other hospitals or using effective recruiting techniques. Montefiore agreed to develop a demonstration program for the recruitment of registered nurses. The target, 350, was reached in three years.

Maurice Hexter, the executive director of Federation, was very doubtful of the affiliation contract. The total budget at Montefiore was around $10 million, and Federation contributed 10 percent of that amount. It was felt that Montefiore's involvement with a city hospital was a diversion of resources from the Jewish community. Later, affiliation contracts became an important source of finances for many voluntary hospitals, including Federation institutions. Cherkasky felt that many of these later affiliation contracts with other hospitals were even

Urbi et Orbi

more flawed than that between the city and Montefiore. Not only were medical concerns separated from administrative affairs, but, in the bargaining process that took place before each contract was signed, many of the features that he regarded as essential for the upgrading of the municipal institutions were lost. The city authorities did not insist, for instance, on following the Montefiore pattern that the house staff at the voluntary hospital be integrated with that at the municipal. Thus, the tradition of separate and unequal care survived, with the better-qualified residents kept at the voluntary institution. Such abuses of the original intent led left-wing critics of the New York hospital system to attack the entire affiliation program as a grab for money and power on the part of the voluntary hospitals, with Cherkasky cast as the *éminence grise* of the plot.

Meanwhile, Cherkasky and Trussell continued as collaborators. With an enormous proportion of health care in the United States paid for as job-related benefits written into union contracts, some unions became interested in influencing the quality of care received by their members. The Teamsters Union, which, with 500,000 members and concerned about the rising cost of hospital care, was investigating the possibility of setting up its own hospital, turned to Trussell in his role at the Columbia University School of Public Health and Administrative Medicine for guidance. A three-part, eight-month sequence was set up: union and management executives attended lectures at Columbia and briefing sessions at Montefiore; at the same time, a survey was undertaken of the hospital care received by a sample group of 300 union members.

The results suggested a high degree of unnecessary surgery. The urgency of better diagnostic services led to the investment of $3,675,000 in a project committed to medical service, research, and guidance for 167,000 union members and their families represented by the Teamsters Joint Council No. 16 and Management Hospitalization Trust Fund. The research phase to be conducted by Columbia provided for continuing samples and evaluations of the quality, amount, type, and costs of medical care received.

A medical advice center was created where members of the union and their families could turn for advice concerning medical and hospital problems. Montefiore Hospital undertook, through a specially created unit, to provide the Teamsters and their families in this program with certain complex specialized diagnostic and treatment procedures such as neurosurgery and cardiac surgery, among others. All these activities were housed in a Teamsters Center at Montefiore. A long-range provision of the contract stipulated that the Teamsters would build at Montefiore a research floor as well as a floor to house the activities of the Center and an additional floor to provide space for a hospital and medical care research team which would use both the research floor for pilot and experimental programs and all of Montefiore as a field laboratory for research into every phase of hospital operations.

Cherkasky was usually a collaborator in his experiments, his strength not in the originality of his ideas but in his ability to put them into practice, to find the resources, to set up the administrative structure, to persuade others to cooperate. He constructed an institution remarkable, not because of any particular program, but because of an ability over a long period of time to sustain a series of experiments in the structure of medical care all designed to tackle the problems of fitting medical care to human and social needs. He developed all the skills of grantsmanship, finding sources of funds in Washington or Albany or New York City.

One of his ventures was a Community Center built by the Associated YMHAs of New York on Montefiore land. The Center and the Hospital collaborated on many ideas: a day care center for the children of nurses and other employees, group activities for discharged psychiatric patients, day care for the frail elderly, a wide spectrum of activities with a medical component for the more vigorous elderly members of the community.

The Board of Trustees, through their social and familial connections, were able to effect an institutional merger that provided the resources for an experiment in nursing.

There was an inherent difficulty in establishing the duties of a nurse in that so many of them could be seen as the services of a personal maid or housekeeper—combing a patient's hair, making a bed. Ward maids and practical nurses could perform the duties that were perceived as demeaning. In many hospitals "team nursing" was introduced as a concept, with the registered nurse directing the work of lesser members of the team.

Cherkasky encountered a nurse who thought differently about the matter. Lydia Hall was vital, charismatic, and opinionated. She came to grips with that first question of nursing, attention to the basic needs of that leaky embarrassing body in which we are all trapped. "If nurses have any area of expertness of their own, then this must be the area of body as body. Bodily care of an intimate nature has long been recognized as belonging to nurses. Bathing, feeding, toileting, dressing, undressing, positioning and moving, as well as maintaining a healthful environment, are encompassed in the area of bodily expertness." Hall vigorously opposed "team nursing." To her, nursing involved all the care required by a patient, and all that care should be given by a registered nurse. To say that any part of that care was less essential than any other diminished the dignity and worth of nursing as a profession.

Cherkasky and Hall found each other at a time when drugs and surgery were making medical care more specific and more intensive and changing the kinds of institutions in which effective care could be given. Prolonged bed rest was perceived as more dangerous than helpful. Fresh air and good food were regarded as part of life, desirable for everybody, not merely the invalid. As the sanitariums, in which these had been the main form of treatment, closed, so did other institutions providing the same formula. "Convalescent homes," in which patients made long and leisurely recoveries, were no longer thought adequate. One of these was the Solomon and Betty Loeb Memorial Home for Convalescents in Elmsford, originally established in honor of Jacob Schiff's parents-in-law. As the Directors, drawn from the same social group as the Montefiore Board, pondered the future of the Home, Cherkasky saw an opportunity, and he enlisted the nurse with as revolutionary an attitude to her profession as he had to his.

The Loeb Board agreed to turn over their future to him and to merge with Montefiore. Using the resources provided by the sale of the Home, and complicated negotiations with reimbursement agencies, Cherkasky built the eighty-bed Loeb Center for Nursing and Rehabilitation as an arena for Hall where her ideas could be put into practice. For eighty patients, who came to Loeb after the most acute phase of their illness had passed, there were forty registered nurses (in three shifts), twenty messenger-attendants, and four ward secretaries. The most remarkable feature of the Center was that it was under the control of nurses. A patient was discharged from Montefiore Hospital and then admitted to Loeb. A physician could recommend admission to Loeb, but the actual decision was made by the nurses in charge. Medical care at Loeb was provided by physicians in the employ of the Center. Hall wanted to get rid of the "jail-like" atmosphere of hospitals: "We stress healing and helping rather than bossing people around." She did not believe that patients could learn to take care of themselves if they were constantly conditioned to passivity by institutional rules. At Loeb, patients were free to set their own pace, to organize their own days. Nurses did not have to wear uniforms.

The Center opened at the end of 1962, with electrified beds responsive to patient touch, washbasins and telephones accessible from wheelchairs, a dining room and a sitting room to encourage movement and socialization. In a few years, studies showed that patients who went through Loeb had a much lower rate of readmission than those who did not. In 1969, Hall died at the age of sixty-three, to be succeeded by her assistant, Genrose Alfano. The Loeb Center continued as a program remarkable for nurse-oriented patient care, and became, and remained, a national model.

Meanwhile, nursing in the main hospital struggled to adjust to the demands of rapidly changing needs. Montefiore was becoming an acute-care institution at a time when the level of patient care in most hospitals was becoming much more intensive. The success of open-heart surgery and the other complex procedures was as much dependent on careful, concentrated nursing as on the surgeons' skills, on monitoring of breathing and heartbeat and body fluids in the first critical hours after the patient left the operating table. The first recovery room opened in the late fifties, where a constant watch was kept as consciousness and feeling returned and the body attempted to adjust to its altered condition.

The profession of nursing was also adjusting. A higher level of education, more solidly based in science, was required for the more sophisticated patient watching, a kind of education too expensive for hospital-based schools to provide, and there was a slow attrition of these as more and more nurses were trained either at community colleges granting associate degrees or at baccalaureate institutions.

The hospitals gradually lost control over nurse training. On the other hand, they became, to a greater and greater degree, the chief employers of nurses. Most health insurance favored hospital care, and nursing care was written in as part of the package. Hospitals found that they could afford to pay better salaries, and families found that their insurance would pay for nursing care in the hospital, not at home. Opportunities for employment outside the hospital shrank, and most nurses were employed by hospitals.

A much more intense level of patient care was also provided by the house staff. In 1961, there were actually two fewer beds at Montefiore Hospital than there had been when it first opened in the Bronx. Then, five residents had sufficed to take care of all the patients. The equivalent number was now 182. Part of the increase was occasioned by changes at Montefiore, but also reflected a general trend in American medicine. Before World War II, more than three quarters of American physicians actively practicing said they were general practitioners or part-time specialists. By 1960, 55 percent were full-time specialists. While it was still possible to go into practice after a year's internship, most of the house staff in a hospital were interested in a longer period of training.

The increased number of house staff and their longer periods of training allowed hospitals to provide more intensive care for patients—and to provide that care twenty-four hours a day, seven days a week. And the trend also helped doctors in practice who knew that when they admitted their patients to a hospital they would be well taken care of. Doctors in practice could handle a larger number of patients in a hospital knowing that they would be cared for at times when the physician in practice could not be present.

Longer periods of training meant that the house staff were older and not willing or able to live on the pittance that had been the prewar norm. With assured sources of funding from insurance and competition for residents, hospitals were able to pay salaries—even salaries that allowed marriage and children. That in turn meant that a different kind of housing was necessary. At Montefiore, the process was assisted by Cherkasky's own memories of house staff activism, and Montefiore was one of the first to start paying house staff salaries that could be considered a living wage. Residents were not prepared to work the nonstop hours that were once demanded of them. As they rebelled, larger numbers were required to provide coverage, since patients persisted in being ill twenty-four hours a day.

The change in the kind of care provided affected the kind of doctors who practiced at Montefiore. In 1950 there were eleven physicians on full-time salaries and a "consulting and visiting staff of 310 internists, surgeons, therapists, dentists and allied professionals." Ten years later there were 64 salaried physicians and 516 attending physicians who were not on salary but had the right to admit their patients. The figures reflect an increase in salaried physicians, a group that was to continue to grow for almost twenty years. The change in the number of attending physicians was actually greater than indicated by the numbers.

The old Hospital for Chronic Diseases was not a place where physicians in private practice admitted many patients. Many of the doctors listed as being on staff rarely came to Montefiore, or came because they were interested in research or public service. They admitted their private patients to other hospitals. The new breed of attendings, many of whom had trained at Montefiore, saw the Hospital as a place to admit their own patients. Just as the young cardiologists brought in by Boas had remained to play a decisive role in the shaping of teaching and research at Montefiore, so the generation of residents trained in the immediate postwar years who went into private practice were also to remain connected to the institution and shape its future. Julius Parker came back from Tennessee and was a founder of the Gastroenterology Service. Harold Rifkin was to become nationally known as an expert in diabetes and would profoundly influence the development of the Loeb Center and the Department of Medicine.

In many hospitals, the attending staff is the single most powerful influence, that force which led to the description of the hospital as "the doctor's workshop." In the old Montefiore, the "consulting and visiting staff," with little financial interest in the place, allowed the Board and the administrator to run the Hospital. They did not grow in numbers or develop an active interest in the Hospital until there was already a comparatively numerous and powerful (since it included the chairmen) salaried staff and a powerful administration. The attending staff at Montefiore was never able to achieve the standing the group enjoyed at other hospitals, a situation for which Cherkasky, rather than history, was often blamed.

Montefiore had all the characteristics of a teaching hospital except an effective affiliation with a medical school. By the late fifties the connection with Columbia existed almost entirely on paper. On the other hand, to become the kind of first-class acute-care institution Cherkasky wanted, to attract the caliber of teachers and residents he wanted, Montefiore needed an affiliation with a medical school.

A partnership between Albert Einstein, the only medical school in the Bronx, and the largest voluntary hospital in the borough, both of them Jewish, appeared obviously desirable. There were obstacles. Einstein was not an independent entity but part of Yeshiva University. Agreements were necessary with both. Dr. Samuel Belkin, the President of Yeshiva, was a dominating personality and an important figure in the foundation of the medical school. The Board of Trustees of Montefiore was still largely drawn from the same German Jewish social class, Reform in religion, as when Jacob Schiff was President. The members of the Boards of both Einstein and Yeshiva were mainly Eastern European and Orthodox. The philosophical differences between the two institutions constantly widened: the one devoted to basic research, the other to social activism, different kinds of people attracted to each. Einstein was firmly in the mainstream of American medical schools: the biochemical sciences the basis of teaching, students drawn from the pool of the most successfully competitive, the role of medicine to diagnose and treat the individual patient. Cherkasky was firmly outside the mainstream, aware that mortality rates in any given community had more to do with jobs and housing and nutrition than with medical care or basic science.

The administrative structure of the Hospital and the College added to the difficulties of bringing them together. At Montefiore, while the Board of Trustees retained ultimate legal power, more and more actual power accumulated with Cherkasky. He ruled with the consent of the governed, but more and more he spoke for Montefiore. The College was truly an academic body, with decisions fought out in arguments in the Faculty Senate. During Cherkasky's tenure at Montefiore, there were six Deans at the College, none of them able to wield the centralized power that he possessed. Indeed, over the years, the belief that the College faculty had in Cherkasky's omnipotence became an important psychological barrier to a close functioning between the institutions. He was seen as such a dominant force that many of the faculty saw any agreement as a yielding of power to him. The natural conflict of interest between the College and the Hospital was often seen as purely a fight with Cherkasky, a perception that his natural arrogance of manner did little to allay.

Fundamental to the conflict was Cherkasky's perception of the role of Montefiore. In a lecture delivered at Massachusetts General Hospital in 1963, he said: "Montefiore Hospital has concluded that it must be prepared to consider carefully any undertaking that seems to have the potential for improving the health and welfare of the people of our community in which its resources, skill, and capacities might play a significant role."

That was an extremely broad view of the definition of a hospital. He listed the programs he thought of as examples of this role—Home Care, the Medical Group, the Family Health Maintenance Demonstration, the Community Center, the Teamsters, Loeb, the affiliation contracts. His vision encompassed more than specific programs. He wanted hospital administrators to become involved in all the great health issues, to fight for social change. He also wanted Montefiore to be an educational center, a place where students came to learn how to develop the skills of social activism. He wanted to train administrators and physicians who could go out into the world and carry his message, to make social instruments of hospitals wherever they happened to be. He wanted Montefiore to be a teaching hospital, but not in the normal sense of the term as a place used by a medical school for bedside teaching. He wanted a hospital that taught, not the normal medical school curriculum, but a set of attitudes and beliefs often at variance with that curriculum. Medical schools normally taught students how to care for the individual sick body. Cherkasky wanted to teach a concern for a whole society, an attitude toward the causes of health and disease of which the medical school curriculum was a small part.

Medical schools were accustomed to being in a dominant position in their relationships with their teaching hospitals, especially as far as setting the curriculum was concerned. The only solution that could have satisfied Cherkasky probably would have been to build his own medical school, a task that was beyond even his ability to find the money and resources and people to implement his ideas, especially when there existed in his borough, a ten-minute car ride away, a medical school dependent upon the sources of private and government money upon which he would have had to draw.

Attempts were made to find another medical school as partner. There were negotiations with Brandeis University. The trustees of Mount Sinai Hospital and Montefiore held months of talks with the aim of achieving joint parenthood of a medical school. The mistrust engendered by Montefiore's championing of unionism and affiliation with city hospitals had not dissipated. The two hospitals had different attitudes toward medicine. Mount Sinai was dominated by one man as much as was Montefiore, but in that case the one man was Gus Levy, the President of the Board of Trustees. Agreement was not likely and foundered over the location of the school—the Bronx or Manhattan.

Formal affiliation of Montefiore and Einstein was announced September 26, 1963, by Belkin and Jacob Schwab, who had succeeded Riesenfeld as President of the Board of Trustees at Montefiore. All of the full-time as well as many of the part-time physicians at the Hospital were to be appointed to the faculty of the College to share in teaching on both undergraduate and graduate levels. Students from the College came in large numbers to Montefiore. The Boards of both remained separate, with a standing committee to oversee the implementation and effective operation of the affiliation.

Between them the two institutions were now responsible for a large portion of the medical care of the Bronx: the beds and outpatient clinics and other programs of the only medical school, the largest and most powerful voluntary hospital, and three municipal hospitals, over 2,600 beds in all. From the beginning the association was strong and lively and profoundly affected all the activities of both places. Over the years, through informal encounters and formal agreements, the working relationships became closer and closer while the marriage remained stormy, each step forward debated in anger and suspicion, often preceded or followed by a step back.

The institution that began as the Montefiore Home for Chronic Invalids became Montefiore Hospital and Medical Center in 1964. The fifties had been spent in the transition of image and policy from a hospital for chronic diseases to an acute-care general hospital. The sixties saw the growth of the new hospital in size and in complexity of purpose.

The expansion of responsibilities required an increase in re-sources: more money, more residents, more teachers, more major divisions, and more subspecialties. In the early part of the decade, Montefiore received an initial grant of $600,000 from the U.S. Public Health Service to establish a new Clinical Research Center. This was the first portion of a total grant of over $4 million to build, equip, and operate a large clinical and basic research facility and to provide basic support for seven years of studies in the fields of cancer, heart disease, surgery, neurosurgery, neurology, psychiatry, and urology. The grant was part of a national program establishing general clinical research centers around the country. Of the thirteen set up, this was the only one in a hospital. All the others were in medical schools. An eighteen-bed patient unit was part of the complex, so that the course of disease could be closely followed at the bedside.

The beloved Daniel Laszlo died, and a Montefiore graduate who had spent the last eight years as head of the Clinical Biophysics Section of the Sloan-Kettering Institute returned as the new Chief of the Division of Neoplastic Diseases. Dr. Leon Hellman was a specialist in steroid metabolism and its relation to cancer.

After Dr. Karl Harpuder retired after twenty-seven years of building up the Department of Physical Medicine and Rehabilitation to national stature, the department was raised to the status of a division with the appointment of Dr. Jerome S. Tobis. Dr. Francis Foldes, an expert on muscle relaxants, was appointed Chief of Anesthesiology.

Montefiore's role as family doctor continued to grow. In 1962 more than 10,000 patients came to the outpatient clinics, and the Medical Group immunized 10,000 people against polio with the Sabin vaccine.

Pediatrics became a division in 1963. Dr. Laurence Finberg came from Johns Hopkins to be chief of the division, which received accreditation for a residency training program from the Council on Medical Education of the AMA. Pediatrics was a rapidly changing specialty. Many of the infectious diseases which had claimed so many children were under control through immunization or the use of antibiotics. As the psychological effects of hospitalization and separation were better understood, the tendency was to keep children out of the hospital whenever possible. The patients in the pediatric beds tended to be only the most seriously ill. Life in the Bronx produced its own hazards. Lead poisoning was frequent, children were hurt in accidents on the crowded streets or fell out of tenement windows, and there were cases of severe malnutrition. Under Finberg's leadership the Division of Pediatrics added enormously to its teaching and research program, strengthening the subspecialties that were becoming more and more important.

The concept of pediatrics was further refined and Montefiore officially recognized another category of patients as defined by age. The adolescents who had always been present on the wards were gathered together in one place. Drs. S. Kenneth Schonberg and Michael Cohen pointed out that it was an expensive move: "There is no economy in grouping teenagers together. When teenagers are spread thinly throughout the hospital, their needs for special facilities, program, and personnel are neither apparent nor obtainable and, therefore, are not addressed. Once having gathered these adolescents together, their requirements become apparent and unavoidable."

Money was not the only difficulty. "Adolescence" was a broad concept. Twelve-year-olds and eighteen-year-olds did not necessarily have much in common—except a capacity to create noise and confusion, especially when their visitors were added to the crowd. They came from many different backgrounds. They were black, Hispanic, white, from every possible social and economic milieu.

Gastrointestinal disease accounted for more than 10 percent of the admissions during the first eleven years, reflecting both the prevalence of such stress-induced conditions as colitis in these stressful years and the frequency of liver disorders among the young drug users of the Bronx. The ability to admit this age group for a more detailed observation and diagnostic work-up than was possible in a doctor's office or outpatient clinic was especially valuable. Suicide was a constantly rising statistic among adolescents, and almost all those who came to the emergency room after an attempt were admitted.

The division was an important center of training for a medical specialty that was just beginning to achieve national recognition. Alumni of the program became directors of adolescent medicine programs in the United States and Canada, and played a role in shaping national and regional public health policies. Out of the inpatient service came an outpatient clinic offering both general and subspecialty care, and the division became responsible for the health-care services at New York City's Spofford Juvenile Detention Center. Out of that relationship came further Montefiore involvement with the prisoners in New York City's jails.

Teaching, research, and expanded services necessitated physical expansion. The thirteen acres of lawns and gardens that surrounded the neat brick buildings, mostly dating from 1912, were quickly covered with buildings, paid for with all kinds of old and new money available to the Hospital.

Existing facilities were converted. According to a story in the house organ, *Tempo*, in the spring of 1964, ongoing construction was "equivalent to building an entire 600-bed hospital from scratch." The capacity of the diagnostic X-ray area was almost doubled by taking down and reinstalling ceilings, by ripping out and relocating walls and rewiring electrical equipment. The hospital's steam-making ability was increased by 30 percent through the installation of a new boiler. Emergency power needs were supplied by three new generators. Two floors of the Van Cortlandt Annex were converted to laboratories and doctors' offices. Six patient floors were added to the Loeb Center, and old courtyards were further diminished as kitchens and storerooms were added.

In the early sixties, Henry Moses, whose tough and demanding intelligence had so influenced the course of Montefiore for forty years, through the Bluestone and Cherkasky eras, died. His widow, Lucy, wanted a fitting memorial. The result was the Research Institute, designed by Philip Johnson, a slim, impressive red brick spire, dominating the skyline and bringing architectural distinction to a neighborhood sorely lacking that commodity. There were seven floors of laboratories, and other floors held a library, a lecture hall, seminar rooms, and a dining room and kitchen—all built at a cost of $4.5 million to the widow, who also provided an endowment fund to provide for the upkeep of the building. There was discussion among staff and Board members about whether the tower should be regarded as a "research institute" with its own semi-autonomous structure, devoted to specific kinds of research, or merely as physical space available to any researchers in need of accommodation. The latter view won. There was never an overall plan for the research carried on in the tower, just a series of laboratories where, over the years, fundamental discoveries occurred.

That May, Montefiore Hospital announced that it would seek to raise almost $35 million to build a new medical center in the Bronx. Thirteen major buildings were listed as "planned or under construction": the new city hospital; the Diagnostic and Treatment Center (the new home of the Medical Group); Maternity Service and Patient Floors; Surgical Facilities; Academic Facility and Beds (the Klau Pavilion); Medical Library and Pathology Laboratories; Student and Faculty Housing; Radiology; Research and Basic Sciences; Ambulatory and Emergency; the Henry L. Moses Research Institute; Montefiore Apartments and Staff Apartments. Not all the plans were accomplished. Community opposition prevented the closing of streets that had been envisioned. The Pill was on the market nationwide and destroyed the dreams of new maternity beds. But by and large the construction program was achieved. The grass and the flowers, cancerous and benign alike, were gone. Montefiore became, instead of Siegfried Wachsman's ideal of German symmetry, a rabbit warren of buildings, differing in shape, in color, in texture, in age. Tunnels connected the buildings underground, and the neighborhood watched as the tentacles spread.

The new Montefiore was built on the rock of health insurance written into job benefits, most of the patients able to pay their bills through Blue Cross, Blue Shield, HIP, or other plans. Some few patients who could not pay could be cared for, but too many non-paying patients could jeopardize the financial basis of the Hospital. A large proportion of the U.S. population had either no health insurance or inadequate coverage.

The mid-sixties brought a national revolution in medical care. Lyndon Johnson was able to push through Congress a flood of social legislation, including, in spite of still bitter opposition from the AMA, a vast extension of medical coverage. It was not national health insurance, the opposition being still too strong. It did provide, however, mechanisms for paying for the care of the elderly (Medicare) and the poor (Medicaid).

Built into the new arrangements were two major flaws. Opposition from the medical establishment ensured that both Medicaid and Medicare were subsidies of the existing system. Both provided that physicians in private practice and hospitals, whether voluntary or for profit, should have their bills paid. In the early years, they were paid on a cost-plus system, in effect allowing hospitals to decide what they should be paid for performing the services they chose to perform. The other basic error was in the structure of Medicaid. Medicare was a federal program, directed at everybody over the age of sixty-five, including middle-class people accustomed to voting and well able to mount lobbying efforts to defend their gains. Medicaid was tied to the welfare system, fragmented among the states, in constant confrontation with that American habit of suspicion of the poor. Each state set its own levels of eligibility and benefits, which in the first years varied from reasonably generous in New York State to pitifully low in the poorer states like Mississippi, which traditionally neglected their own low-income populations.

In 1966, the operating expenses of Montefiore Hospital and Medical Center were $19,246,194. The equivalent figure ten years later was $135,094,496. The cost of each bed for a day of patient occupancy had gone from $85 to $206. The sources of those dollars had changed profoundly. In 1966, philanthropy contributed $959,862 of the $19 million budget. Ten years later, the budget was almost six times as much. The philanthropic contribution was not even twice as large. "Patient, Blue Cross and Other Insurance" provided $133,121,977.

Cherkasky was quick to realize that Medicaid and Medicare and other Great Society programs were a bonanza for medicine and its institutions. He also sensed that free access to the pot of gold would not last forever. In these early days hospitals were free to expand services, knowing that they would be reimbursed. The impact was seen in the growth curve of Montefiore's budget: total costs ran around $4 million in 1951; ten years later the total was somewhat over $10 million; by 1971, over $75 million; by 1981, around $230 million. These vast amounts of money came from government or from government-regulated third-party payers. The philanthropic contribution increased very little over thirty years; from about $1 million to about $1.5 million. That meant, in effect, that the philanthropic contribution became a very small part of the budget, diminishing the power of the Board of Trustees.

Such sums of money required a high level of professional expertise in their management, and the funds did not come unencumbered. With them arrived a huge and complicated network of regulation. An even higher degree of skill was required to comply with the legalities and, at the same time, make sure that the hospital was free to fulfill chosen missions. During these same years, medicine became more and more sophisticated, less and less open to decisions from non-professionals, and as the task of hospital administration became so complex, the Board of Trustees was forced to rely more and more upon the judgments of the man they had chosen.

The role of the Board of Trustees had changed rapidly and in response to unrelated developments. The money donated, while a smaller and smaller fraction of the operating budget, was still an important ingredient in the funding of new construction or special programs. Involvement in day-to-day hospital business became less and less. Until after World War II, the white-gloved finger of a female Trustee was accustomed to testing the furniture for dust. Unionization and professionalization took the details of housekeeping out of the bounds of Board concern. Until after World War II, as long as the majority of the patients were objects of charity, admitted for long-term care, the Trustees passed on the applicants for admission. At the new Montefiore, the physicians made the decisions about who was to be admitted. Most had some form of insurance. The Social Service Department searched for funds for those in need. As regulations, imposed by government, insurance carriers, and accreditation agencies, came to control more and more hospital activities, the Board had very little discretionary or decision-making power. The Trustees retained, however, full legal responsibility for the institution, a heavy burden as doctors and their hospitals became more and more frequently the object of public dissatisfaction and private suits. And as hospitals became bigger and bigger business, the Trustees' skills in business and law increased in value.

In some ways their role did not change. The members of the Board remained as concerned about medical care for the very poor as their grandfathers had been; they were also as interested in the general problems of public health, especially the health of the people of New York City. Many of them were political and social conservatives; in matters of health care, they were still willing to be radical. They agreed that their institution should become involved with the city hospitals and with the drug-ridden poverty of the South Bronx.

Many saw Cherkasky as dominating his Board of Trustees. His power was achieved by the expenditure of a great deal of energy on the process of persuasion. He spent endless hours talking with individual members on the telephone, meeting with them over breakfast or lunch or dinner, in discussions with the various committees. He drew upon their knowledge when he needed it, he used their business, financial, and political contacts, and he endlessly explained his important moves to them. Board meetings, which were moved back downtown to that bastion of the German Jewish establishment, the Harmonie Club, became more and more pro forma. There were few debates or contested votes because he had spent so much time convincing them before the meeting. He did not risk his leadership by bringing matters to a vote before he had laid the groundwork and was sure of support. Some Board members chafed at the degree of control and direction; others enjoyed the feeling of being caught up in an adventure.

In the mid-sixties, Edmund Rosenthal, whose family had been involved with Montefiore over generations, became Chairman of the Board. Riesenfeld and Schwab had been older than Cherkasky, father figures delighted with the bright young man. Rosenthal was approximately the same age as Cherkasky. The two developed an abiding friendship that outlasted their official connections. Gentle of manner, literate, cultivated, with an abiding interest in health care, reflected in his service to the Menninger Foundation, Rosenthal presided over the Board during Montefiore's most explosive period of expansion, bringing to bear on that hectic era a concerned and caring mind and heart and a civilized humor.

Elliott Hurwitt died suddenly in the mid-sixties. The particular interest of the chief of a department in any hospital strongly determines the direction of teaching, research, and patient care within the department. The new Chief of Surgery, Marvin Gliedman, was especially concerned with transplants and brought with him people such as Dr. Frank Veith, who shared his interest. The first kidney transplant at Montefiore was done in 1967 on Mrs. Dora Russek, a forty-three-year-old Bronx housewife suffering from an infection which was destroying both her kidneys. While awaiting a transplant, she was being treated as an outpatient in the Renal Dialysis Unit by the machines which cleansed the blood of those whose kidneys were not functioning. Dr. Robert Soberman was in charge of the Kidney Service and the Dialysis Unit. Mrs. Russek was at home when the call came that there was a kidney available. She rushed to the Hospital, where the kidney was being kept alive on the heart-lung machine and Blood Bank technicians were lining up appropriate donors. Gliedman, Veith, and Dr. Selwyn Freed removed both the patient's kidneys and inserted the transplant. By the time Mrs. Russek was discharged three weeks later, a second patient had received a transplant.

A Major Organ Transplant Center opened with three dialysis machines, used to maintain fifteen patients, and a four-bed Intensive Care Unit, able to accommodate fifty kidney transplants a year. The full-time staff included, as well as the four physicians especially involved, seventeen nurses, four renal fellows, a psychiatrist, a social service worker, residents in medicine, surgery, and urology, and other auxiliary personnel. The unit was planned for lung, liver, and heart transplants "when initiation of programs in these areas becomes practicable." That day was not to arrive quickly. Although kidney transplants quickly achieved a high level of success, other forms of transplants remained rare. The immunosuppressive drugs used to control the body's immune mechanism, responsible for the rejection of transplanted organs, impaired the body's ability to fight infection and heal wounds.

In 1968, Leiter retired as Chief of Medicine, and after an interregnum with Harold Rifkin as Acting Chief, he was succeeded by David Hamerman, who had trained under Leiter and, admiring his mentor's style and approach to medicine, modeled much of his behavior on that of the older man. Thus, the two largest departments at Montefiore were led by two new men just when the resources that flowed from Medicaid and Medicare were becoming abundantly available.

Both Hamerman and Gliedman set about broadening and deepening their departments, adding people with new skills and new specialties. Gliedman found a department where the chief was essentially a practicing surgeon who also held the job of chief, most of the surgery done by the senior surgeons and most of the surgeons using other hospitals to admit patients. Gliedman changed all that. Although he continued to do some surgery, he spent most of his time organizing and running the department. When he arrived, there was only one salaried surgeon on staff—and two more at Morrisania. He brought five salaried people with him and gradually built this up to thirty-six full-time salaried surgeons, basically young people, though with established reputations, with an interest in both patient care and research. They came from two groups: successful private practitioners who decided they would like to come on salary and residents who wanted to stay on after graduation. Gliedman was proud that so many members of his department achieved national or international recognition: "Dr. Clarence Schein (at Montefiore since the forties) was a world authority on biliary tract diseases; Dr. Scott Boley an internationally known individual in pediatric surgery; Dr. Veith has become an enormously well-known transplant surgeon and vascular surgeon."

Surgery benefited from the way in which the reimbursement systems worked. They all favored surgery as a method of treatment—and they all favored in-bed treatment as opposed to ambulatory care. In the early years of Medicaid and Medicare, there were few constraints on the way in which the money could be spent: hospitals were free to buy new equipment, hire new people, add residency positions and training programs. Gliedman was able to give his people what they wanted—money and space.

Gliedman saw his role as nurturing other people, handing over to them even those areas of surgery that were his own area of expertise. When Veith became Director of the Transplant Service, Gliedman restricted himself to pancreatic transplants. On the other hand, he also believed that as chief he had to continue to operate or lose the respect of other surgeons.

Under Finberg and Gliedman, the Departments of Pediatrics and Surgery worked together to develop a program in pediatric surgery. The success of surgery in infants and children is dependent on an understanding of their physiology, and surgical care was not separated from general pediatric care. Every child undergoing surgery was also under the care of a pediatrician, and in many cases psychological support was also included for the parents.

In all general hospitals, the Department of Medicine is the single most important clinical department, with the largest number of patients covering the widest age distribution and with the broadest range of diseases. Indeed, as long as chronic diseases were the only business of Montefiore, the Department of Medicine almost was the Hospital, with surgery one of the auxiliary services provided.

With 293 beds—and 94 at Morrisania—this was still the largest service, with the largest number of attending staff, with the most varied number of subspecialties. In a teaching hospital, the interests of the subspecialists were expressed in research and therefore this department produced the most research on the most subjects and was in constant need of research space.

David Hamerman made profound changes in the structure of the department when he took over. His first move was to convert the rotating internships during which interns had moved from service to service, acquiring a broad experience. Now most medical school graduates wanted to specialize. Hamerman set up straight internships, with graduates going immediately into the field in which they wanted to specialize. These training courses were more attractive to the brighter students. Four years after he took over, there were 357 candidates for 42 internships in internal medicine. At the same time that he was encouraging specialization, Hamerman was also aware of the cry for primary-care physicians, for general practitioners, for family doctors, and he worked closely with the Residency Program in Social Medicine and later the Department of Family Medicine in developing their training, allowing the residents in those programs to spend part of their time on the wards as well as in community health centers, in learning the concepts taught in social medicine as well as the more traditional curriculum. A general medical clinic was established in the Outpatient Department where house officers spent time each week seeing their own panels of patients.

Bluestone and Cherkasky had brought physicians in on full-time salaries partly because of their own opposition to fee-for-service medicine. Teaching hospitals in general began to add salaried staff for the same reason as medical schools: to strengthen teaching and research, allowing people to devote all their time to these activities instead of being distracted by the demands of practice. When Hamerman took the job, the only subspecialties headed by full-time people were cardiology and hematology. He proceeded to bring in salaried people to head and staff many more subspecialties, so that by 1972 the department, as well as internal medicine, included: allergy, cardiology, dermatology, diabetes, endocrine, experimental immunohematology, gastroenterology, geriatrics, hematology, infectious diseases, pulmonary diseases, renal, and rheumatology.

In the meantime, the borough in which the Hospital stood, particularly the South Bronx, was so profoundly affected by the forces that were destroying the inner cities of the United States that it became the national symbol of urban decay. Most of the private physicians had long since left the area, and with the emergency rooms and outpatient clinics of the city hospitals unable to deal satisfactorily with the day-to-day medical problems of thousands of families, medical care was dangerously inadequate. The other conditions of the area were as bad as the medical care: decaying tenements, burned-out stores, garbage-strewn streets, stripped automobiles, a high rate of unemployment, addiction, school dropouts, and teenage pregnancy—reflecting a low level of hope in a community where the average age was twenty-four. One of those who tried to bring hope was Harold Wise, who had a grounding in community medicine before he came to the Bronx. After graduation from Toronto University Medical School, and then going to San Francisco for an internship at the Kaiser Foundation Hospital, that pioneer of pre-paid group practice, he spent six months in Saskatchewan, where the cooperative movement flourished, working in a cooperative community clinic, before returning to Kaiser for a residency in internal medicine. From there he came to Montefiore for a further two years of residency, becoming Chief Resident in Medicine and then Director of Ambulatory Services and Home Care at Morrisania. Cherkasky described him as possessing "a tough, critical analytical mind," and "an enduring and seemingly endless commitment to the task of developing new mechanisms, new workers, and new relationships to help change the miserably inadequate health-care services available to all people in this country, and especially the kind of care given to those who have suffered the most—the blacks and the Puerto Ricans, the Chicanos and the poor whites."

Wise went into the streets to find out what the people who

lived there wanted and what Montefiore could do to help. He knocked on doors and listened to groups gathered in apartments. These people wanted health care for themselves and their families and they wanted it in an atmosphere where they were treated with respect, something different from the overcrowded, understaffed, and underequipped clinics of the city hospitals. More than health care of any kind, however, more than any other services, they wanted jobs.

Physicians in private practice had fled the South Bronx for good reasons—the fires, the muggings, the break-ins in search of drugs. The traditional model of American medical practice could not survive in this battleground even if Cherkasky and Wise had thought it useful or suitable. They did not: ". . . we decided that the most appropriate model would be a well-organized group practice unit located in the heart of the deprived area, in one main center and two satellite centers, to be staffed by health professionals who for the most part would not be living in the community." Montefiore assumed responsibility for the program and provided all of the backup support in addition to essential consultative and diagnostic resources.

Provided with a grant of $2.2 million from the Office of Economic Opportunity, and directed jointly by Montefiore and Morrisania, the Martin Luther King, Jr., Health Center was planned to serve 8,000 families. An old multistory building at 170th Street and Third Avenue was remodeled. At a satellite on Bathgate Avenue, 1,500 families registered by the fall of 1967 and the first thirty family health workers graduated. Eight doctors and four public health nurses offered internal medicine, obstetrics and gynecology, pediatrics, and minor surgery.

The position of family health worker filled several needs. One was to provide jobs for neighborhood people. The locally recruited workers went through a twenty-four-week training program. Most were women. (Throughout its history, the Center attracted more women than men as both patients and staff.) Each one, supervised by a public health nurse, cared for between twenty and forty families, making home visits to check vital signs, bathe patients, change dressings, give enemas, check diets, and make sure that patients were following through with treatments. They also tried to help with housing and welfare dilemmas.

These were not the only jobs provided. In a little over two years, more than two hundred local people were trained as rehabilitation aides, lab assistants, record room personnel, and operating room technicians. Some graduates of the in-house training program went on to full-time college or training programs. One of the family health workers, Deloris Smith, the mother of seven children, obtained a master's degree in public health and ultimately became the director of the project, by then a multimillion-dollar enterprise.

The aim was to provide the best possible scientific medical care, and one essential ingredient for that was continuity. American medicine was following the twin roads of specialization and fragmentation. Family doctors were disappearing. The typical middle-class suburban family used the services of several doctors: an obstetrician-gynecologist, a pediatrician, an internist, surgeons, or other specialists easily available for referral. The poor who used the clinics in the public hospitals received even more piecemeal care. The Center was to do things differently. Each patient, or family, was assigned to a team made up of a doctor, a public health nurse, and a family health care worker, with other professionals called in as needed. The patient visited the same team each time, with the family health worker assuring continuity between visits.

The Center was a success. By 1971, 390 people from the neighborhood had gone through training programs. There were 33,000 registered patients and that year a quarter of a million services were provided. The infant mortality rate for the babies delivered by women cared for at the Center was one third that of the general rate in the area. National recognition was implicit in the fact that the Center received almost 30 percent of the OEO funds available for such programs.

There was one continuing running sore. In spite of all the careful preparation, there was constant conflict and misunderstanding between the Community Advisory Board (composed of residents of the area) and the Hospital administrators. Cherkasky was aware of the insoluble nature of this battle: "Despite the clear understanding of the advisory nature of the board, there has been constant pressure by the board for involvement in administrative and policy-making decisions not envisioned in such a relationship. There was a notion that no matter how advisory its nature, the board really should be the final authority with regard to hiring, firing, and program development."

The Advisory Board was affected by the hostility between blacks and Puerto Ricans in the area and by the fact that the Martin Luther King, Jr., Health Center was almost the only functioning social institution in an area of fragmentation, instability, and crime and violence. There was a rapid changeover in population in the area which the Center actually assisted. The people who received training and found jobs tended to move out of the area to live, even if they commuted back to the workplace.

Montefiore administrators continued to meet and talk with community groups, discussing structure and organization, the ultimate aim to turn over control to the community. This was the great bone of contention, to be fought over month after month, year after year. Viewpoints differed about timing. Hospital officials saw community control as a long-term goal far in the future, believing that the only way to establish financial stability and medical excellence was for Montefiore to assume, and for some considerable time retain, responsibility. The neighborhood people wanted change fast.

This was the sixties: the United States was in turmoil, long hot summers the norm, the cities in flames, riots a recurrent theme, the lid off the melting pot, and all the dissatisfactions of society boiling over. The administrators found themselves the objects of violent vituperation at community meetings, "black power" and "community control" the rallying cries. Cherkasky long remembered the angry young black man who told him that he would rather destroy the program than have it controlled by the white establishment.

The Great Society provided other grants for experiment. Another health care center opened, the Montefiore-Morrisania Division of the Comprehensive Child Care Project, funded by a grant from the Children's Bureau of the Department of Health, Education, and Welfare to the Albert Einstein College of Medicine. It was one of two programs set up by the College to care for children in Bronx poverty pockets, to provide an alternative to the emergency room/outpatient clinic care that was the only form of treatment available. Long waiting times were to be eliminated. Visits were by appointment except in emergencies, and every effort was made to see patients on time. The same team approach was used as at the Montefiore-sponsored centers: each child or family assigned to a pediatrician, a public health nurse, and a social worker. The staff planned to teach mothers about immunizations, nutrition, child development, and so on. The Director, who arrived from basic research in the labs at Albert Einstein, was Dr. Mutya San Agustin, a Filipino pediatrician who became so intrigued with the problems of providing good ambulatory care that she never went back to test tubes. Small, vital, and energetic, she devoted her time to lecturing, hectoring, and attempting to move an immovable system.

Lead poisoning was endemic to the Bronx through the combination of gasoline-laden air and the lead-based paint that peels off the walls and windowsills and ceilings of old apartments. Two medical students from Albert Einstein, working through the Project, began a lead poisoning screening program as part of their field work experience for a course in community medicine. Bill Rhodes and Bob Young began by spending a spring evening drawing blood samples from forty-nine children in three buildings in the South Bronx. They followed up with a one-day program, and as a result, three children were registered in the Project for treatment. The two students recruited fifteen more College students, who in turn rounded up 110 highschoolers, who were paid by the Community Council of Greater New York to visit apartment houses to check for lead-based paints and to draw blood and urine samples from all the children living there. One side effect of the screening program was that 130 children were brought into the Project.

Students were the foot soldiers of the revolution of the sixties. Out of school for the summers, they flocked South for voter registration drives, to Washington for demonstrations, and to the ghettos of the big cities. In the summer of 1967 more than sixty medical, dental, and nursing students came from over thirty colleges and universities to join the Student Health Project of the South Bronx, another OEO-funded program, sponsored jointly by Montefiore and Albert Einstein. They worked in emergency rooms, health centers, Headstart classrooms, community psychiatry programs, and outpatient departments.

Conflict between a medical school and a teaching hospital is probably an unavoidable ingredient of the relationship. In most cases, the medical school is the stronger and more prestigious of the institutions. In this case, Montefiore was older, independent, and with its own deep philosophy and traditions, and was not Einstein's first or only teaching affiliate.

The 1,400-bed Bronx Municipal Hospital Center was the first hospital to which the students of the new medical school were sent. In the sixties, as New York City extended its program of upgrading city hospitals, a request was made of Einstein to come to the aid of the old Lincoln Hospital in the South Bronx. Einstein provided staff in pediatrics and, after the passage of the Community Health Act in 1963, in psychiatry. The venture was not without hazards. Students and staff from Einstein, exposed to both the appalling physical inadequacies of this shabbiest of city hospitals and the grinding poverty in which many of the patients normally lived, reacted with horror. And there were profound differences of approach. Many of the members of the Department of Psychiatry at Einstein were trained and functioned in a traditional psychoanalytic mode; those interested in setting up the storefront community health centers for which money was now available from the federal government were interested in quite a different approach. The same kinds of differences—personal and philosophical—appeared when the Department of Medicine sent people to Lincoln. Community activists in the area demanded their share of power at Lincoln. Thus a medical school which had pinned its faith to basic science and began life with a mission of serving Jewish students found itself willy-nilly involved in the street battles of the Bronx of the sixties and trying to deal with students and programs in teaching hospitals with wildly differing atmospheres.

Community activists, on the other hand, often saw more unity than actually existed. As the borough became less and less Jewish, there was growing resentment of these two powerful Jewish institutions, with frequent references to the "Montefiore-Einstein Empire," often at times of great tension and enmity between the two institutions.

Events were to bring them closer. Einstein had on its faculty many physicians who were interested in caring for their own patients. Accommodations were lacking. Not only were city hospitals looked down upon by people who could afford to pay for their own care, either through insurance or out of pocket, but the rules of city hospitals did not allow doctors to admit private patients. The College authorities decided to build a hospital for the use of faculty physicians and their patients. Unfortunately, it was built without proper attention to Blue Cross and its rules. By this time, Blue Cross had developed reimbursement rates related to hospital size, complexity of treatment, and provision of services to the community such as emergency rooms and outpatient departments. Montefiore, with almost 800 beds, large training programs, outpatient services, and community involvement, had a large financial base and fulfilled the requirements for top reimbursement rates, which were over $100 a day at that time.

The College Hospital, on the other hand, too small with only 375 beds to be financially viable and lacking some of the community services that Blue Cross required, received only $74 a day, even though the care provided by the sophisticated medical school staff was both complex and expensive. The result was that the College Hospital ran a deficit, which had to be made up by the College. In time, the drainage of money threatened the existence of the College.

The answer was found in an arrangement with Montefiore. Blue Cross agreed that if the larger hospital and the smaller were combined in one full-service institution, the higher reimbursement rate would apply to both, and on January 1, 1969, Montefiore assumed operational responsibility for the College Hospital. (The Dean of the College at the time was Harry Gordon, a pediatrician who had studied pathology under David Marine at Montefiore.)

Other economies were possible with data processing, including inventory, payroll, and medical statistics centralized at Montefiore along with many accounting, purchasing, and personnel functions. Cherkasky hoped that ultimately there would be more important savings, that the coming together of the two hospitals would be the beginning of a rational plan of health care for the entire borough: "If the medical community is ever to provide compassionate, high-quality hospital and medical care to the entire Bronx, it cannot expend resources, money, space, and personnel in duplication of services and non-productive activities which serve only institutional pride or ambition." He hoped that "those programs which can best be carried out at the College Hospital are carried out there, and those which can best be carried out at Montefiore are carried out there." And he felt that the dream which had first begun with the affiliation with Columbia in 1916 was on the way to fulfillment: "We here always felt that Montefiore's own ability to lead the way in hospital care was dependent upon a sound, vital relationship with an outstanding college of medicine. We believe now that our unity with the Hospital of the Albert Einstein College of Medicine will fix the Montefiore complex more firmly into the heart of the medical school and that, in this way, we will together be able to more effectively meet our goals in patient care, education, and research."

C H A P T E R

17

Hospital, Community, and College

The Montefiore reaching out to the community had the same intense interest in scientific research closely related to patient care as it had in the past. Theodore Spaet, M.D., headed a Division of Hematology constantly discovering new properties in blood. Dr. Norman Trieger, who succeeded David Tanchester as head of dentistry in 1970, strongly objected to the repair-shop school of thought that pervaded his craft. He wanted his residents to pursue basic research and to collaborate closely with other physicians and surgeons. Work that had begun with children with cleft palates developed into the Cranio-Facial Center, where dentists, plastic surgeons, ophthalmologists and neurologists worked together to rebuild faces distorted by congenital defects, disease, or accident. Paul Henkind, M.D., who came to head ophthalmology, developed a staff and an outstanding program devoted to research, especially in the area of macular degeneration, a common difficulty of old age. Leopold Koss, M.D., followed Zimmerman in pathology. His specialty was cytology, the study of cells, an interest which flowered in a study sponsored by the National Cancer Institute in the detection of endometrial carcinoma, the most common cancer of the female genital tract. Since 1945 the Headache Unit has helped 30,000 people afflicted with this most common of human ills, developing both new remedies and new understandings. Under Elliot Weitzman, the Department of Neurology became involved with another of the most frequent of ailments, setting up a Sleep-Wake Disorders Unit, which proved to have, as well as serious scientific significance, immense popular appeal.

In 1971 the Medical Center's income was $75,230,283. Research and Grant Program expenditures totaled $17,312,473. Montefiore was now responsible for 1,504 beds: 719 in the main hospital, 80 in the Loeb Center, 374 at Einstein, and 331 at Morrisania. All the institutions together had 321,110 outpatient visits and 180,617 emergency room visits. The Martin Luther King, Jr., Health Center had 40,000 patients registered. Four hundred and sixty-two residents and 352 medical students served and studied patients in the varied locations. There were 463 physicians on salary and 5,508 "administrative, technical and other employees."

In many respects, Montefiore reflected what was happening to hospitals all over the United States. Large and complex institutions were typical of a health-care industry that had become the third-largest employer in the country. Decisions concerning health-care issues were likely to be affected by pressure from groups anxious to preserve their own interests in an important sector of the economy.

Medicaid and Medicare poured money into the existing system with very few controls over the way in which it was spent, and one result was an enormous increase in the cost of care. From 1966 to 1969 the average rise in the Consumer Price Index was 12.9 percent. For medical care as a whole it was 21.4 percent; for physicians' fees, 20.9 percent, while the daily cost of a hospital bed was an incredible 52.4 percent. Montefiore had a relatively small deficit: $610,909. Other hospitals in urban areas serving larger numbers of the uninsured or less astute about finances teetered on the edge of bankruptcy. Magazines and newspapers during the seventies were given to running stories about the "crisis in health care." The fuss was about the cost of health care, which by the end of the decade approached 10 percent of the Gross National Product. The United States was spending a greater percentage of its wealth on health care than any other developed country while providing coverage for a smaller proportion of its population.

"Cost containment" became the popular political issue of health care in the seventies. Washington had a special interest. In 1965 health-care costs accounted for 4.4 percent of the federal budget. Eight years later, the figure was 11.3 percent. The answer was regulation, and a flood of legislation in the early seventies created organizations and rules whose purpose was to control cost and sometimes quality as well. The latter purpose may have occasionally been accomplished. The first most certainly not.

Federal attempts to control costs were often ineffectual because of inflationary factors built into other federal legislation. One particular law of these years led—as an unforeseen side effect—to vast new expenditures. By 1972, nationwide about 9,000 people suffering from some form of kidney failure were having their lives prolonged by the use of kidney dialysis machines. The cost was formidable and usually not covered by insurance. In response to pleas from patients and their families, Congress agreed that Medicare would pay the cost of dialysis for everyone.

States and localities also had a vested interest in health-care costs. Some responded by further slashing benefits or raising eligibility requirements. New York State, with a more liberal tradition, was less likely to take that route. Moreover, in New York City, with its huge system of municipal hospitals and with seven medical schools and their related institutions (also intertwined with the municipal system), there was probably a concentration of the instruments and interests of medical care unique in the world. There was also a longer tradition of attempts at planning for health care than in most parts of the country. As early as 1964, New York State began to control capital expenditures of hospitals and nursing homes. In 1971, it began setting hospital rates and throughout the seventies was better able to curb costs than most states.

In the sixties the rising costs of providing service altered the structure of the Montefiore Medical Group, affected not only by the increasing expense of its own services, but also by the precipitous upward climb of inpatient care. Hospitals were reimbursed on a per diem basis, theoretically the cost of maintaining one patient in one bed for one day. This figure was calculated by combining all the costs of running the hospital—heat and light and food and wages and so on. The actual cost of caring for a patient who walks in for an office visit and leaves in half an hour is obviously less than for one who stays overnight in bed. The lumping together of all the expenses to arrive at the per diem figure made the expenses of the Group or any other kind of outpatient care appear to be higher than they actually were. The Health Insurance Plan of New York, also hard hit by rising costs, refused to pay the Group the rates necessary for solvency. In 1970, the Group was forced to leave HIP, give up the essential idea of prepaid service, and ask patients to pay for each visit. Enough of them were loyal to the Group, and also carried insurance that could help pay the cost, to continue their visits. Then another piece of legislation from Washington enabled the Group to again offer guaranteed prepaid coverage. The War on Poverty had encouraged alternative forms of health-care delivery for the poor. During the seventies, Washington encouraged more economical methods for the already insured with the passage of legislation aimed at the establishment and nurture of prepaid group practices, renamed HMOs. Employers with twenty-five or more employees were required to offer them the opportunity to join an HMO as an alternative to regular health insurance, if they lived in an area served by a certified HMO. The first HMO in New York State under the new law was set up by Blue Cross and Blue Shield of Greater New York and called the Community Health Plan of Greater New York. The plan contracted with the Montefiore Medical Group to provide services to members who lived in the Bronx, Manhattan above 174th Street, and Westchester below the Cross Westchester Expressway. Benefits included full coverage for physician services, for 365 days of semiprivate hospital care, for maternity care, diagnostic tests, well-baby care, immunizations, and ambulance services as well as benefits for private duty nursing and emergency care outside the Montefiore area.

The Medical Group was now back in the business of prepaid practice, and with a large clientele of young families. This was a different generation from the original Group patients. They did not expect house calls. On the other hand, many of them had grown up without the experience of their own physician. They had received their medical care from hospital clinics and emergency rooms. Shirley Grossman, still Medical Director of the Group, explained that part of staff responsibility was training these families how to use the service now available to them —to come by appointment, to consult a pediatrician by telephone.

Montefiore had begun as the most paternalistic of institutions. No doubt had crossed the minds of the original Trustees about their inborn right to make decisions on life-and-death matters. The original patients had not been a particularly docile group. The paying patients of the seventies were as demanding. One administrator was given to worrying that standards in the Hospital would fall off when the Jewish grandmothers were no longer around to complain. The ethnic composition of the patients had changed greatly. As long as the Hospital for Chronic Diseases existed a very large proportion of the patients were Jewish, since many of them were referred by Jewish agencies. Most of the doctors were also Jewish, a circumstance that made for easier understanding and rapport.

By the seventies, the patients came from all the many ethnic groups of the Bronx, although there was still a high proportion of elderly Jewish patients. Many of the doctors were still Jewish, with enough of a mixture to lead to the sight of an Indian resident from Madras learning Yiddish so that he could communicate with his elderly patients. The nurses had never had a large Jewish component. Nursing had now become the same kind of profession for the upwardly mobile black woman that it had once been for the Southern white woman; workers were either black, Spanish, Yugoslavian, or Albanian.

There were now deep cultural differences between physicians and patients, between physicians and nurses, between nurses and patients, adding to the stresses of delivering care. And there were profound differences between Montefiore and the Bronx, a borough where political activism and ethnic hostility were endemic. Montefiore and Einstein were seen together and separately as rich, powerful institutions in an area becoming poorer and poorer, and perception on the part of others as Jewish added an abrasive bitterness that affected attitudes on both sides.

Many programs now had as one of their goals the bridging of this gap between institution and client. For Social Medicine this was often the primary aim. George Silver left Montefiore in 1965 to become a Deputy Assistant Under Secretary with the Department of Health, Education, and Welfare. He was not replaced for four years. All departments at the Hospital were in a constant process of change and adaptation, dependent upon the state of scientific knowledge and technology, patient demand, and the interests of each chairman. Social Medicine remained the most ambiguous, a discipline whose content or direction was the least predetermined, any aspect of the relationship between medicine and society an appropriate field for study or active intervention. Comparison with other institutions was not especially helpful in the search for definition. Other hospitals which set up similar departments and labeled them Social Medicine or Community Health usually expected no more than administration of the ambulatory-care clinics, social change rarely written in as an accepted bureaucratic goal.

The third Chief of Social Medicine at Montefiore, comfortable with societies in the process of revolution, took the department off on a pathway different from any trodden before. Dr. Victor Sidel created a new kind of department, exploring the wide world, not in the manner of the visiting academic making careful statistical comparisons, but in the guise of a latter-day Marco Polo bringing back startling information of curious inventions from a China hidden from American view for twenty years.

Sidel came to Montefiore from Boston, where he was Chief of Preventive Medicine and Community Health at Massachusetts General. At the same time he was active in Physicians for Social Responsibility, the organization founded in 1962 to fight against nuclear proliferation and against the Vietnam War and Agent Orange. This latter interest resulted, two years after he arrived at Montefiore, in an invitation from the Chinese Medical Association, and he became a member of the first group of American physicians to visit China after the United States recognized that country. He brought with him news of the success of the Chinese government in dealing with public health problems. One technique he adapted to the needs of the Bronx: community residents were trained in the skills of Chinese barefoot doctors, although shoes were necessary for protection in the garbage-strewn streets. Isolation and loneliness were two of the greatest hazards to health in the Bronx of the seventies. The number of Jewish residents had been declining for thirty years. The children who fled to the suburbs left behind a residue of elderly people, more and more confined to their apartments by ill health or fear. Equally alone were many of the young Hispanic mothers, new to the area, cut off from social contacts by unfamiliarity with the language and customs. Sidel's department sought out representatives of both groups, as well as the Irish families in the area, and trained them to take blood pressures, do simple first aid, and spot obvious health problems among their neighbors. More than a hundred of these workers were trained, and they helped the young mothers find companionship and medical resources for their children, helped the elderly keep track of their medications and shop for each other, and helped the lonely rediscover a sense of community.

The only direct clinical services provided by Sidel's department were through the Methadone Maintenance Treatment Program, funded by the Office of Substance Abuse Services of the New York City Department of Health. A Child Care Health

Project funded by the Robert Wood Johnson Foundation was administered by the department with the intention of improving health care in day care centers. Nancy Dubler, a lawyer, conducted a series of seminars on legal and ethical issues in the delivery of health care in prisons and edited a new publication, *The Journal of Prison Health*. Dubler also joined with a philosopher, Richard Roelofs, to conduct a series of explorations of legal and ethical issues within the Hospital, questions about a patient's right to refuse treatment, the whole problem of the meaning of "informed consent," and the problems of providing intensive care in a neonatal unit. A Bioethics Committee was formed to provide a broadly representative forum for discussion of legal and ethical issues and to make recommendations to the Director. One of the early case studies was that of an adult who refused a blood transfusion on religious grounds. Sidel, Roelofs, and Dubler also led the Committee on Research on Human Subjects.

From the beginning Montefiore had dealt with patients whose ill health was the result of the conditions under which they worked: the nineteenth-century painters with lead poisoning, the young women who contracted tuberculosis in garment industry sweatshops. In 1979, the U.S. Department of Labor funded the department to place medical students with union locals, to learn about health problems from the point of view of the workers and then put this knowledge to use. At the same time the Department of Health, Education, and Welfare backed a program to make occupational health part of the medical school curriculum. The Department of Community Health at the College under Herbert Lukashok as acting chief collaborated with Sidel on all these projects.

Roberto Belmar, M.D., a university professor and Deputy Director of the National Health Service in Chile under the Allende government, fled the country in 1973 and became one of that long line of political refugees who contributed at Montefiore. With his encouragement, the Department of Social Medicine became heavily involved in Latin America. Health education projects were set up in Colombia. At the request of the United Nations Fund for Population Activities, Belmar participated in the development of a Maternal and Child Program for Guatemala and an Assessment of Maternal and Child Health Needs for the Republic of Mexico, as well as advising the Nicaraguan government on medical programs. There was a constant interchange of visitors between the department, other countries, and international health organizations.

This was a very different department from that which Silver had run—and it did not include all the programs that could be classed as "social medicine." The truth was that while other hospitals or medical schools had departments called Social Medicine or Community Health or some variant, Montefiore itself was, under Cherkasky, one large Department of Social Medicine, even while the department that theoretically had that subject as its main agenda continued to function. Thus, the whole hospital became a social medicine laboratory. There was no attempt to organize "social medicine" activities administratively segregated from the rest of the Hospital. Programs were placed in whatever niche seemed appropriate, run by any administrator who seemed capable. The programs which had made up Bluestone's original Department of Social Medicine drifted away and achieved autonomous life. Other programs took root and flourished in whatever corner of the administrative structure offered a haven.

Cherkasky's only criterion seemed to be effectiveness. Over the years, administrators tried to bring some semblance of order, without much success, frequently frustrated in their efforts at pruning because the people who ran the kind of programs that Cherkasky especially liked, frequently were found to have easier access to his office than others less favored.

One of the structural oddities that resulted was the Residency Program in Social Medicine, which was administratively quite separate from the department of the same name. Harold Wise devised this training program with David Kindig, a young resident who had come out of the Midwest and a life devoted to laboratory research to find a new direction in the South Bronx. Wise and Kindig wanted to solve two problems: the staffing of the Martin Luther King, Jr., Health Center and the provision of appropriate training for physicians who wanted to care for the people of the inner cities.

Kindig and Wise wanted a training program that dealt with a broad spectrum of questions. They wanted to teach physicians to deal with children and their families in their own environment; to deal with healthy as well as sick people; to learn an awareness of cultural differences; to see "medical care" as a much broader term than as it was usually used; to learn to work in collaboration with other health professionals. The Residency Program in Social Medicine began in 1970. Residents could train in internal medicine or pediatrics. A family medicine track was added in 1973. All the residents spent their first seven months in full-time traditional inpatient rotations, taking care of patients in the beds at Montefiore. At the end of that time, each one was paired with another in the same specialty at the same level of training. This allowed two of these trainees to assume the Hospital responsibilities of one full-time resident in the traditional program. The other half of their time was spent as members of an interdisciplinary team at Martin Luther King.

Hospitals are, on the whole, hierarchical and authoritarian, residency programs usually run strictly at the discretion of the chief of the department. This was an oddity among residencies in that it was not part of a department—the Director never had the awe-inspiring authority of a chief—and chiefs of other departments could strongly affect the fate of the program. In addition, Wise and Kindig built in a large degree of democracy. Residents took part in the management of the Residency Program in Social Medicine, they argued out the curriculum, they evaluated the staff, and each class took part in the interview and recruitment process to select the following year's class.

As well as planning a different kind of training, Wise and Kindig wanted to attract a different kind of person as a resident. American physicians were still overwhelmingly white males. The Residency Program in Social Medicine set out to attract candidates who were more closely connected to the patients of the South Bronx by language and ethnic origin. Wise and Kindig themselves fell into that category of residents who came to Montefiore because they wanted to change society and the practice of medicine. Their Residency Program attracted a concentration of such people, and the process of each class recruiting for the following year ensured a continuation of the same type of person, which, in turn, generated an atmosphere that was rarely calm. Heated discussion was the norm: on issues of politics, of racism, of sexism, within and without the Hospital.

Community activists demanded certain kinds of health care. Soon after New York State passed a law legalizing abortion up to twenty-four weeks of pregnancy, members of the Bronx Women's Liberation Group approached Montefiore and demanded that the Medical Center provide an ambulatory abortion service for the women of the neighborhood or for those who came from other areas. At first the administration resisted, maintaining that the service was being provided at a satellite about five miles away. That was not good enough for the women, and a committee was formed representing the Liberation Group, administrators, and the heads of Gynecology and Social Medicine. At first there was considerable mutual suspicion, but after several months of discussion an agreement was reached whereby a separate, nonprofit corporation was set up to operate the Bronx Community Abortion Center with a board of directors of whom five represented the Hospital and four the community. The Montefiore Board of Trustees guaranteed a loan from a local bank of $250,000 to buy equipment, furnishings, and supplies. The Hospital leased a one-story building two blocks away to house the Center.

The state and city Departments of Health approved the plans; the Hospital provided medical staff and administrative supervision. Lay staff were trained as counselors. Patients were examined, counseled, and prepared for abortion at the first visit, with the actual abortion scheduled for the next day, so that the women had a chance to reconsider. The Center was open from Tuesday through Saturday and most holidays. The standard Medicaid fee was charged. Patients who had no means of payment were referred to a municipal hospital. In five years, 13,778 abortions were performed. For the first three years the Center operated at a loss and then began to break even financially. All patients were provided with contraceptive advice. Those who came back for three or more abortions (a small number) were referred for further counseling.

Like their nineteenth-century counterparts, the physicians were dealing with a poor immigrant population with all the differences of language, culture, and education. Misunderstandings were frequent. One young patient was the seventeen-month-old son of a Puerto Rican father and a mother from El Salvador. When the little boy was brought to the pediatric clinic at Morrisania, he was seen by three physicians, who recognized the symptoms of rickets and told the parents that he was well but needed vitamin D and would be admitted to Montefiore Hospital. But when the parents saw the machines to which he would be connected, they became frightened. In spite of explanations from the house staff, the nurses, and the administrator on duty, the parents took their child home.

That might have been the end of the matter, but Dr. Peter Andrus, an intern in social medicine, was determined that the child should be appropriately treated and, together with a social worker, set out to establish contact with the parents. He learned that they were taking the little boy to a podiatrist in the South Bronx. Andrus called the podiatrist, who agreed to set up a meeting with the parents in his office. There, away from the frightening atmosphere of the hospital, in a place where they felt comfortable and in command of the situation, the parents allowed Andrus to administer medication to the child and set up a plan for future out-of-hospital treatment.

The city of New York asked for help in dealing with other citizens. In 1973, the city contracted with Montefiore for health care at Rikers Island, the city prison where those awaiting trial or sentenced to less than a year were held. On a normal day, there were about 7,500 people in the New York City Correctional System. During a two-week period in June 1975, a survey was done of all 1,420 prisoners admitted to the system. Three quarters of them were under thirty years of age, 57 percent were black, 26 percent were Hispanic, and 17 percent white. Forty-one percent reported previous drug use. More than one quarter reported an illness themselves, and three fifths were diagnosed as having at least one illness. The most commonly diagnosed conditions were drug abuse, psychiatric disorders, trauma, and alcohol abuse. Visitors to the program were often startled by the contrast between the Montefiore clinics, freshly painted and clean, and the dirt that seemed to pervade the prison as a whole.

The brief period of incarceration provided its own frustrations for the professionals, cutting periods of treatment short. Referrals were made for follow-up care, but these were difficult to sustain. Some of the anticipated difficulties did not occur: female nurses were able to work in the program. A high percentage of female physicians were attracted to the program because of the regular hours. Administrators found a high rate of "burn-out" among the professionals because of the tensions and frustrations inherent in the situation, and tours of duty were deliberately limited.

The inmates at Spofford included both the most vicious of young criminals and children whose main problem was not having a place to sleep. They showed a range of problems: those, like malnutrition, that were the result of poverty, and a high percentage of trauma and drug abuse. They also suffered from the beatings and rapes that they endured from other inmates or from the guards.

Both the adult and juvenile populations bore the stigmata of medical neglect. They had received little dental care or correction of chronic conditions; their immunization records were poor. Caring for them forced the physicians and nurses to become involved in other aspects of prison administration. A prisoner with diabetes, for instance, was provided with insulin, but control of diet was difficult: all coffee came pre-sugared. Many of the juvenile offenders, being black or Hispanic, were lactose-intolerant, being unable, like most of the world's non-white population over the age of infancy, to digest milk. The meals at Spofford were planned, however, according to Department of Agriculture guidelines, to include large amounts of milk and milk products, which caused many of the young prisoners to suffer from chronic diarrhea.

The Social Services Department changed to meet the needs of the new kinds of communities. In 1970, while the staff remained mostly female, a man became Director of Social Services. Gerald Beallor reflected the trend toward a psychiatric orientation in social work, coming from a position as the Director of Psychiatric Social Services at Coney Island Hospital in Brooklyn and with his own private practice in family counseling and psychotherapy. Social workers were, of course, always concerned with the psyche of the client. With many of the physical needs met by government agencies—through food stamps and welfare payments and rent subsidies—the role of the social worker changed often to the frustrating one of guide through the red tape.

The problems were the same dilemmas that had always troubled patients: working parents who needed someone to stay with a sick child, suspected cases of child abuse, a constant visitor to the emergency room too terrified to accept the surgery that would end her pain. There were changes. One was in the growing number of elderly patients. They tended to have complicated physical conditions with a galaxy of symptoms, to recover slowly, to stay longer in the hospital, and to require more care when they went home. Often they lived alone or with partners who were themselves elderly and frail. A growing proportion returned not to their own homes but to nursing homes, and the care in these homes varied from excellent to totally inadequate. "Discharge Planning Committees," representing Social Service, Home Care, nursing and medical staff, became an important part of the hospital routine, making sure that all patients would be cared for after they left Montefiore.

The population around Montefiore was becoming older. Around 22 percent were over sixty-five as compared to a national average of 10 percent. Research focused on the specific difficulties of the elderly. Alfred Weiner, M.D., and Irwin Gerber, Ph.D., conducted a five-year study of the medical, social, and psychological repercussions of bereavement on older people. At the same time, they tried to estimate the effectiveness of a brief period of psychotherapy in helping patients deal with the effects of the death of a spouse. Members of the Medical

Group were asked to participate, and more than 90 percent of those who were invited agreed.

The researchers found that in the first fifteen months after the death of a spouse, 66 percent more of the bereaved visited their doctors for major illness than did the non-bereaved, and there were equally significant increases in the number of general medications taken, the number of mood-altering drugs taken, and the number of complaints of general malaise. The study also showed that those who received psychotherapy, with the chance to talk about feelings, pain and sorrow, and love and guilt and anger, visited doctors less, used less medication of any kind, and in general felt physically better.

Finding a suitable place for sick elderly patients was a major problem, not only for the Department of Social Services but for the institution as a whole. For some of the most helpless a link was forged with the Beth Abraham Hospital, a "skilled nursing facility" by New York State reimbursement definition and providing a high level of medical and nursing care to patients who resembled the old Montefiore population in the severity of their chronic and probably incurable illnesses.

Beth Abraham lay about halfway between Montefiore and Einstein. Founded in the early twenties by a group of Orthodox rabbis' wives as a traditional nursing home, it was being trans- formed into a modern, medically sophisticated hospital under the direction of its energetic Director, William Adelman. He approached Cherkasky for help, and there developed between them a personal and professional friendship that resulted in an often informal but effective sharing of resources. Members of the Montefiore Board and their friends were persuaded by Cherkasky to accept seats on the Beth Abraham Board, which began to meet at the Harmonie Club immediately before the Montefiore Trustees gathered together. Solid working relation- ships were established with other nursing homes. Home care was still an important part of the program for discharged patients. The Montefiore experience had influenced legislators to include home care as a Medicare benefit, and during the seventies there was a gradual extension and inclusion of home care by other reimbursement agencies. Isadore Rossman, a physician who had worked with Daniel Laszlo, and now Director of Home Care and a world authority on the subject, decided to bring some of his homebound chronically ill patients back to the hospital once or twice a week. They were transported in wheelchairs, and received physiotherapy and occupational therapy. They were able to borrow books from the hospital library, have their hair done by hospital beauticians, and they visited together as a group for tea and cookies. This program gave the patients, who often led quiet, isolated lives, the opportunity to get out of their houses and see something of other people. The Community Center ran a day care program for the frail elderly of the community, again giving them a chance to meet others and socialize. Both programs also provided a brief respite to family members who normally cared for the patients.

The rapid growth of the elderly population, combined with the continuing disintegration of the Bronx community, meant that none of these measures was sufficient. A decision was made that Montefiore should sponsor a nursing home. Plans were drawn up, local and state approval obtained, arrangements for financing made. At the last moment, the government of New York State decided that no more nursing home beds should be provided in the Bronx and approval was withdrawn.

The patients in Montefiore needed new space as much as discharged patients did. Attempts to serve the community did not always meet with community approval, especially when construction was involved. An addition was made to the limited operating room facilities when Dr. Harold Laufman, Director of Montefiore's Institute for Surgical Studies and Chairman of the Committee on Operating Room Environment of the American College of Surgeons, was able to persuade fifteen companies to contribute over $250,000 in grants for experimental projects and $110,000 in equipment in order to put together an ideal surgical environment. Control systems were installed that allowed each surgical team to adjust lighting and ventilation to the specific needs of each operation, and careful records were kept over time to establish standards for future operating room design.

Unfortunately, that future kept receding. Much of the plant

was out of date. The building erected in 1912 still stood, in need of constant repair, the wiring totally inadequate to the demands of the high technology of the seventies. Montefiore had been one of the first hospitals to eliminate long wards. Now the four-bed rooms built in the fifties looked crowded, uncomfortable, and shabby; the corridors were crowded with patients on their way to operating rooms, food carts, and visitors. The number of operating rooms was inadequate. Recovery room space was in even shorter supply. Occasionally, surgeons were forced to hold a patient on the operating table because there was no space in the recovery room.

The administration drew up plans for building. Hospital construction, however, required permission from layers and layers of bureaucracy, from local community boards to Albany and Washington. With public funding had come intense public regulation.

The first hurdle was the immediate neighborhood. Construction had been more or less continuous during the Cherkasky reign. Local householders resented the dust and noise. The construction of North Central Bronx Hospital on land donated to the city by Montefiore aroused particular ire. The Green House, the Victorian clapboard in which generations of administrators lived, was torn down. The last stretch of lawns and gardens disappeared with the excavation of a hole several stories deep as the base for a seventeen-story tower. Neighbors worried that a new building would bring more traffic, more ambulance sirens, and a different kind of population. Like most people in the Bronx, they were scared as they watched the fires and the devastation approach from the south, convinced that any change could only be for the worst.

To the residents of other parts of the Bronx, Montefiore appeared to be one of those malignant forces drawing population and jobs out of the South Bronx. The building of North Central Bronx on Montefiore land, joined to Montefiore by bridges, became a subject of bitter community dispute. The construction of North Central Bronx (NCB) meant the closing of Fordham and Morrisania Hospitals. Health care was one of the popular radical causes. The expansion of Montefiore was seen as the growth of another "medical empire" against the best interests of the poor and helpless. When Montefiore first offered the city land on which to build a replacement for Morrisania, the offer was gladly accepted. The proposed site offered convenience: the Montefiore medical staff, serving the municipal hospital under the affiliation contract, could walk easily between the two institutions, making for easy supervision and consultations; patients could easily be transferred from one to the other.

By the time the North Central Bronx Hospital was ready to open in the late seventies, the political and community atmosphere had changed. The South Bronx was still in a process of further disintegration. Acres and acres of buildings had burned. Neighborhoods were in chaos, held hostage by the terror of crime and arson. The inadequate number of jobs that had existed in the area was shrinking daily. At one time, the city government had agreed to close and replace both Morrisania and Fordham. Faced with growing financial problems, plans were changed. Both hospitals were to be closed; only one new hospital was built. The closing of Morrisania meant the removal of one of the few stable institutions which brought money and jobs into an area that was rapidly collapsing. The formal opening ceremonies of the new hospital were awash in waves of hatred as community groups assailed those responsible for the closing of the old ones. The assembled officials of both hospitals were asked to pray for "the souls of those who died because the emergency rooms at Fordham and Morrisania were closed."

North Central Bronx was an attractive building. The cafeteria on the top floor offered an unparalleled view and quickly became known as "Windows on the Bronx." The police also came to appreciate the view since it allowed for surveillance of acres of the rooftops of the Bronx. Glen Neilson, an ex-policeman who had been chief of security at Fordham and had transferred to NCB, found the design of the building helped his job. Montefiore's haphazard growth and spilling over into neighborhood houses had created a multiplicity of entrances that made effective patrolling impossible. NCB, planned at a time when security was uppermost in the minds of the urban architect, had limited exits and entrances. There was also none of the shabbiness associated with city hospitals. This one was sleek and shining. In compliance with a city law that mandated that a certain percentage of construction money be spent on artwork, the walls were colorfully attractive. Gone also were the long wards traditionally associated with municipal hospitals. The rooms were small, and this in itself, it seemed to Neilson, affected behavior. There was less violence, fewer arguments, less smuggling and dealing in drugs or other contraband.

Bob Bloom had also transferred from Morrisania. The task was easier here with a new building and with the journey from Montefiore a walk along a corridor. There were still problems, legal, bureaucratic, and physical, with the transfer of patients. There were still the problems caused by the division of authority. There were still hostilities. If a Jewish doctor and a black nurse did not see eye to eye, each was likely to account for the other's actions with references to ethnic origin. In spite of the problems, NCB quickly achieved the highest level of occupancy of all the city-owned hospitals.

Mutya San Agustin, who had established the modus operandi of the Comprehensive Health Care Center, took over the outpatient department at NCB and created something quite different from the fragmented, episodic care that patients received in the clinics of the traditional public hospital. At NCB each patient who came in to the clinics was assigned to a primary-care team consisting of a physician (either an internist or a pediatrician), a nurse practitioner, a social worker, and a resident. The whole team functioned as a family doctor, assessing the patient's overall health status, home environment, and total needs. At each visit the patient was cared for by the same team.

Believing that the answer to discontinuity of care lay in not blaming the patient but in devising systems that encouraged continuity, San Agustin was constantly inventive. Wanting to ensure that new babies were seen regularly by a pediatrician, she introduced pregnant women to a pediatrician at around the sixth or seventh month for a discussion of the coming baby and any other children. Studies showed that 80 percent of these mothers followed through and took their babies, once they arrived, to the pediatrician for regular visits.

The obstetrical beds at NCB were popular, with an occupancy rate of more than 100 percent. (Obstetrical statistics are different from other occupancy rates since the patient may actually spend more time in the labor and delivery rooms than in the ward.) The delivery of babies in the United States followed divergent paths in the seventies and eighties. There was a great increase in cesarean deliveries in hospitals while at the same time there was an increase in births at home or in more home-like settings within hospitals. The obstetrical service at NCB followed the second trend. In 1982, 2,700 babies were born there, 90 percent of them delivered by midwives. NCB had the lowest cesarean rate of any hospital in New York City and one of the lowest in the country. The midwives not only delivered babies; they advised mothers before and after birth on caring for themselves and their children.

The most profound organizational change of the seventies came with the attempts to develop a closer relationship between the College of Medicine and the Hospital, with representatives of the two arguing, bargaining, and fiercely disputing the details of the match. At the heart of the quarrel were two different attitudes toward the education of physicians.

To Cherkasky, his rebellion against the American medical system and his attempts at change could be successful only if he could educate the young physicians who would take over the leadership of the revolution.

He saw the attraction of medical school affiliation, but he was not prepared, for the purpose of achieving those desirable ends, to sacrifice his hospital's autonomy, to accept the somewhat subservient position normal in the teaching hospital–medical school relationship. He wanted the place where patient care was carried out to be as important an influence on a physician-in-training as the academic setting, and he wanted social concerns to be as important as science in that training. He believed that "the purpose of the medical school is, firstly, to provide an educational process which will best prepare a physician to carry out all the responsibilities which properly fall to a physician in his goal of protecting and promoting the public health; secondly to increase knowledge and do other things. What has happened is that the increasing of knowledge and doing other things have become the primary purpose and there has been a kind of unspoken—or maybe spoken—notion that if you make good enough scientists out of them, they will become good enough doctors."

As he saw it, only part of the education of a physician took place in a medical school. Equally important was the time spent in the hospital, learning through interactions with patients and with the other people who worked there. Students, interns, and residents learned through their experiences on the floors of Montefiore, through the teaching of the full-time and voluntary staff there. They learned also in the different settings provided in the complex: the emergency room, the outpatient clinics, the health centers in other parts of the Bronx and Westchester. The skills of patient care, social attitudes, and community needs were all part of the agenda.

In 1974 a new Dean, Ephraim Friedman, an ophthalmologist, arrived at the College. He was to stay for nine years, nine years of painful argument out of which came fundamental agreements.

As desirable as some kind of Montefiore-Einstein union might appear, there were severe limitations on what could be accomplished. Einstein was a highly successful medical school educationally and financially. It was not, however, independent, and the only patient-care facility it actually owned (HAECOM) was under lease to Montefiore. The Bronx Municipal Hospital Center (BMHC), its first teaching hospital, was at the mercy of New York City's financial fortunes, which for much of the seventies teetered on the edge of bankruptcy. Montefiore was a financially stable hospital with a series of linkages of varying degrees of formality or legal enforceability with other institutions, many of its most distinctive activities dependent on a constant process of renegotiation of contracts with governments or foundations or, in the case of HAECOM, with the College itself.

The decision was made in the early years of Friedman's tenure that the clinical departments could be unified, to take advantage of all the varied settings with which each partner had contact, for the purpose of educating future physicians and providing service to a large proportion of the people of the Bronx. The process of putting this decision into practice was long, often bitter, and constantly illustrated the reality of the differences in philosophy and practice of College and Hospital.

The first unified department was Surgery under Marvin Gliedman, Montefiore's Chairman of Surgery. The result was a sprawling conglomerate with almost 800 beds in four hospitals: 298 at Montefiore, 158 at HAECOM, 100 at NCB, and 240 at BMHC. Patients going from operating rooms to beds were not the only responsibility of this gargantuan department: in a typical year there were 187,000 visitors who required surgery in the emergency rooms of Montefiore, NCB, and BMHC. (HAECOM still had no emergency room.) Outpatient visits added up to 52,603 in general surgery, 625 cardiothoracic procedures, 7,233 in plastic surgery, 25,864 in orthopedics, 42,000 ear, nose, and throat treatments, 2,230 in neurosurgery, and 9,221 genitourinary procedures.

By 1980, all the surgical specialties were unified across both campuses: the Department of Orthopedic Surgery under Edward T. Habermann; and Neurosurgery under Hugh Wisoff. Berish Strauch headed the Division of Plastic and Reconstructive Surgery, and Robert W. M. Frater the Division of Cardiothoracic Surgery.

Interns and residents originally won a foothold in hospitals because they were a cheap way of providing care for patients. In return for food, lodging, uniforms, and education, they were prepared to work endless hours. By the seventies they had managed to limit their hours and were receiving salaries sufficient to support not only themselves but spouses and children. They had become an expensive form of help. Hospitals began to look for alternatives.

The Department of Surgery was concerned about another issue. The United States was notorious for an overproduction of surgeons and a rate of surgery above that in comparable nations. Gliedman did not want to add to the surplus. On the other hand, a certain number of residents were necessary to take care of the growing number of surgical and emergency room patients. Three physician's assistants arrived from Duke University trained to take patient histories, do physical examinations, order routine lab tests, and perform minor surgery. Dr. Richard Rosen coordinated their work, and soon he and Clara Vanderbilt, one of the trio from Duke, were running a training program for physician's assistants at Montefiore.

The unification of the department was accomplished during a period of rapid change and development in the art of surgery. New developments in surgery were dependent on a multitude of factors: new drugs, new machines, better anesthesia, better aftercare. One kind of surgery was especially dependent on one of the oldest of scientific instruments, the microscope. In microsurgery, in which Dr. Berish Strauch was a pioneer, the surgeons worked, not by looking directly at the patient, but by looking through a microscope that enlarged one tiny portion of the body from eight to twenty times. They manipulated blood vessels and nerves less than one millimeter in diameter, sewing tissues so delicate that a touch could bruise, with sutures almost invisible to the naked eye. Mastery of the skill took practice. In 1974, Strauch, with Dr. Avron Daniller, led a two-day workshop to teach twenty-four other surgeons these demanding methods, each participant provided with a microscope, sutures, and instruments. For one full day they worked on the repair of small nerves, using the sciatic nerve from a rabbit. The next day they learned to repair the aorta of a rat.

Microsurgery promised much. "For the first time," said Strauch, "we can attempt to reimplant a hand or finger that has been amputated in an accident, because we can see to work on the tiny blood vessels without injuring them and, therefore, we can reestablish circulation through the severed appendage." Soon, reimplantment was a common reality. Montefiore became one of the two centers (Bellevue was the other) in New York City to which accident victims and their severed arms or legs or toes or fingers, carefully wrapped in ice and plastic, were rushed. Helicopters set down on the nearby Reservoir Park, unloading their freight from surrounding counties and adding another element of noise to which community residents objected.

Reattaching a limb required time and a team of experts. When a railroad worker was hit by a five-ton automatic spike driver, his leg was almost completely severed between the knee and the ankle. His leg was saved after nineteen hours in the operating room by a team of eleven that included an orthopedic surgeon to deal with the broken bones, two reconstructive plastic surgeons, a vascular surgeon, two reconstructive plastic fellows, two residents, an anesthesiologist, and two nurses.

Techniques developed by Frank Veith, the Chief of Vascular Surgery, were important in transplants and reimplantation, in both of which the repair or rejoining of veins or arteries was important. With Dr. Seymour Sprayregen, professor of radiology, he headed a team devoted to the saving of legs threatened by amputation. Many patients with diabetes or heart problems suffered from poor circulation, which ultimately could result in gangrene. With a combination of X-ray techniques that allowed for accurate estimates of the site and degree of blockage, and surgical methods that included bypasses around the blockage created from either the patient's own vein or an artificial graft material, the team probably saved 1,000 legs in eight years.

They built on long traditions of vascular surgery at Montefiore, where there had always been many patients with these problems. So did the Cardiothoracic Service, which worked closely with the Cardiology Service. A senior medical cardiologist attended each patient before and after surgery and was present in the operating room. The anesthesiologists and nurses in the operating and recovery rooms were specialists in the care of the cardiac surgical patient, and part of that tradition of cardiology at Montefiore that stretched back to Boas and before.

By 1970, 1,000 patients had been equipped with pacemakers. One hundred of these later died and 400 needed the device only temporarily. This left 500 with permanent implants, and since the pacemakers were powered by batteries and there was no way to predict when these batteries might fail, patients had to be checked regularly to make sure that the batteries were retaining their power. For the first eighteen months, the checks were made every six months. After that, the checks were more frequent until, to avoid any risk, the unit was replaced sometime between twenty-four and thirty months.

The whole process was time-consuming for patients and staff. Seymour Furman went to work with Bryan Parker, the Yorkshireman in charge of the electronics lab, to devise a more convenient form of testing. They came up with a system using the telephone. Each patient was given a small, portable transmitter. When the time came for a check, he or she went to a telephone and called the catheterization lab. The telephone was placed on the transmitting device, and the patient grasped two metal electrodes attached to the apparatus in both hands. The rate at which the pacemaker was operating was transmitted to the lab. The whole procedure took only a minute or two and could be done as often as once a week. Not only was the method easier for everybody; it was possible to keep such close track of the battery life that replacements could be postponed and patients saved from additional surgical procedures. Ten years later the number of pacemaker implants approached 2,500, all requiring follow-up care.

The Cardiac Catheterization Laboratory, which housed the pacemaker project, was always outgrowing its quarters. Around 1960, the patient load was increasing at the rate of 25 percent a year. New expanded space had just been occupied in 1971 when, as Dr. Doris Escher, who had remained in charge of the program, explained, "all statistics soared and the space crunch was renewed." Coronary bypass surgery, the replacement of clogged vessels with veins taken from other parts of the body, was big business, and cardiac catheterization was the essential diagnostic tool in the form of angiography: an opaque fluid was fed through the catheter into the arteries and the amount of blockage could then be studied. While occasional national studies cast some doubt on the need for the total quantity of bypass operations performed in the United States, procedures proved so popular that when Dr. James Scheuer arrived as the new Chief of Cardiology, plans were immediately laid for constructing a second floor on top of the Telephone Building to provide more space. No sooner was that floor complete than plans to convert the entire cardiac catheterization unit to an updated, essentially operative suite were announced. The result by the late seventies was that the area had four operative suites, two of them equipped for high-quality X-ray diagnosis. One room was used for fluoroscopy, pacemaker implants, and electrophysiology studies, another for minor surgery and pacemaker changes. In support of these units were clean and dirty utility rooms, a five-patient stretcher and recovery area with emergency support, locker and changing areas for all staff, and facilities for developing and viewing films. In the catheterization and angiography room, the patient was laid on a table that had side-to-side, head-to-foot, and up-and-down motion and could be swung readily 90 degrees from right to left on its base.

In the same year in which Gliedman took over this surgical empire, David Kindig, who had been working for the federal government in Washington, came back to the Bronx to become Director of Montefiore Hospital and Medical Center. The new title of President was created for Cherkasky.

Kindig's own interest was in community medicine, but he found that the further working out of the relationship with the College occupied a major portion of his time.

The country's economic troubles had deeply affected the cities. New York City was approaching bankruptcy and was forced to cut back on many services, including the city hospitals. Much of the College's teaching program was based at BMHC, and Kindig found that there was pressure for HAECOM to fill some of the gaps left at BMHC by cutbacks in city funds. Under the terms of the lease, Kindig could make decisions about HAECOM. On the other hand, much of what happened there depended on decisions by the College faculty.

In 1979 the lease under which Montefiore ran the College Hospital expired. There had always been a group among the faculty which resented Montefiore—or Cherkasky—power. They persuaded the College not to renew the lease. For six months, the College attempted to administer the Hospital. All the conditions which had plagued the Hospital in the sixties recurred. Also, it was simply too small to be financially viable. The reimbursement agencies reduced their per diem payments. Again, the Hospital began losing vast amounts of money, threatening the College itself with a fatal hemorrhage of dollars. The only answer was to again allow Montefiore to run the Hospital.

Montefiore's first female chairman was appointed to head a new Department of Clinical Sciences in 1980. Rosalyn Yalow had assisted in the first nuclear medicine experiment. Since then she had worked in the laboratories of the Bronx Veterans Administration Hospital, where her work in developing radioimmunoassay techniques led to a Nobel Prize, the first American woman to receive the prize in science and only the second woman in history to receive it in medicine. Trained in nuclear physics, she was chiefly interested in the application of her discoveries in clinical medicine and the encouragement of young physicians to take up careers in research.

Radioimmunoassay, the tracking of minute quantities of substances through the body, was used in the diagnosis of obscure causes of retardation, in the study of the passage of insulin, and even in solving several cases of murder. Yalow was persuaded by Cherkasky to come to Gun Hill Road but, loyal to the Veterans Hospital, which had supported her research for so long, insisted on spending half time there.

By 1982, almost a third of the first-year medical students in the country were women. The rate of change had been rapid; only ten years before the figure was 6 percent. The restrictions placed on women in medicine had lasted so long, however, that even if this one third ratio of medical students continued until 1990, only 8 percent of the 600,000 physicians practicing in the

United States would be women. There were the beginnings of an advance in the faculties of medical schools, but again, from such a low starting point that women were still clustered on the bottom rungs of the ladder. The Department of Psychiatry was unified under the chairmanship of Herman van Praag, a native of the Netherlands, whose interests reflected more the basic science research interests of the school than the clinical interests of Montefiore. He came from the post of head of the Department of Psychiatry at the Academic Hospital of the State University of Utrecht. A specialist in biological psychiatry, whose research was in the field of the biological determinants of abnormal behavior, van Praag brought a different set of skills and a different direction to psychiatry at Montefiore.

Pediatrics was perhaps the specialty which had changed most since the turn of the century, when infectious diseases were the greatest threats to infants and children and the hold on life of any baby was so tenuous. Indeed, much of the increase in life expectancy came from the reduction in infant mortality. Now the average baby born at full term could look forward to a healthy infancy and childhood. Pediatricians began to pay more attention to the far ends of the spectrum, to adolescents and premature infants.

Since World War II, there had been a gradual building up of knowledge about the physiology of premature babies and techniques of surgery and transfusion to deal with some of the anomalies. Other factors fed into the interest in the newborn. Many new medical techniques—monitoring devices, microsurgery—could be adapted to the care of these tiny patients. Teenage pregnancy was of epidemic proportions, and these young mothers tended to produce small infants.

Among adolescents, the great killers were not diseases but automobile accidents, suicide, and drugs. The Division of Adolescent Medicine was probably as good a place as any to view the connection between disease and social conditions. In one paper, three physicians on the staff (Iris F. Litt, S. Kenneth Schonberg, and Michael Cohen) wrote about society and one particular organ of the body: "The liver, unfortunately, bears

many of the scars of the social, psychological, and biological
revolutions that are simultaneously occurring in adolescents
today. As a major organ of metabolism, it is adversely affected
by the drugs and toxins that teenagers use; by the hormonal
changes of adolescence; . . . and even by changes in sexual
patterns as reflected in gonorrheal perihepatitis and the effects of
oral contraceptives." One of these three, Michael Cohen, became Chairman of the Unified Department of Pediatrics.

The Bronx was becoming an area of the old and the young. Of
the Bronx's 1,400,000 people, 500,000 lived in the northeast
Bronx around the College and the Bronx Muncipal Hospital
Center, and of the half million, a third were between the ages of
six and twenty. The streets of the northwest Bronx around
Montefiore were equally full of children, and to serve them the
Department of Pediatrics offered services that ranged from the
thirty-five-bed pediatric inpatient facility at the College Hospital, which was basically a diagnostic and therapeutic referral
service for seriously ill children from across the country and
even from other countries, to the tertiary-level neonatal center
for twenty-five sick infants at BMHC, and 330 other inpatient
beds. Just as important were all the ambulatory settings. Three
of the hospitals had busy emergency rooms and outpatient
clinics. In addition, there was the Comprehensive Family Care
Center, a freestanding program operated by the College offering
medical, dental, nursing, social service, nutrition, and speech
and hearing services to 8,000 people, mostly low-income; the
Rose F. Kennedy Center for Research in Mental Retardation
and Human Development, with its major activity the diagnosis
and treatment of handicapped children; and the Comprehensive
Health Care Center, the heir of the programs begun in the sixties,
and now under Dr. Stanley E. Harris, a group practice giving
quality care to children and adults and working closely with the
schools in the area.

Protracted negotiations took place over the appointment of
the chief of the largest and most important department, Medicine. The College enthusiastically supported the candidacy of
Dr. Louis Sherwood from the Michael Reese Hospital in

Chicago. The endless discussions between Cherkasky and his chairmen centered on the question of whether Sherwood fully supported or understood the concepts of unification and regionalization. On the other hand, since Gliedman was seen as a Montefiore person, there was felt to be a certain obligation to honor the wishes of the College. Sherwood had a profound interest and a distinguished career in research in the clinical disorders of calcium metabolism and the structure, function, and secretion of polypeptide hormones. In his writings, he emphasized the role of a department chairman in fostering research. After his arrival he structured the department in such a way that his own position was almost the only unifying force: "The Department of Medicine of the two campuses is a single academic department under one chairman. However, the general internal medicine residency training programs are separate and applicants may apply to both or either. . . . Each campus has a vice-chairman of the Department of Medicine responsible for the day-to-day operation of the patient care and house staff training programs."

Separateness was emphasized: "The Department of Medicine . . . is one of the largest in the country. With five constituent hospitals on two campuses, containing over 3,000 beds, of which over 800 are devoted to internal medicine, and operating two major house staff training programs."

The department at Montefiore encompassed eleven divisions: the Blood Bank under Morton Spivak, M.D.; Dermatology under Peter Burk, M.D.; Emergency Medical Services under Anthony Mayer, M.D.; Endocrinology and Diabetes under Martin Surks, M.D.; Gastroenterology under Leslie Bernstein, M.D.; Hematology under Theodore Spaet, M.D.; Immunohematology under Parviz Lalezari, M.D.; Infectious Diseases under Neal Steigbigel, M.D.; Pulmonary Medicine under M. Henry Williams, Jr., M.D.; Renal Medicine under Norman Bank, M.D.; and Rheumatology under Arthur Grayzel, M.D. (While men still ran the department, about half of the first-year residents were now women.)

At Montefiore, the medical training program included 200

beds on the Klau Pavilion, 25 beds for pulmonary medicine and pulmonary intensive care, 35 cancer beds, and over 40 intensive-care beds. Five interns had managed to care for 650 patients in 1915. In 1981, for the thirty-six patients on each floor of Klau there were four interns and two residents as well as clinical clerks and subinterns from the Medical School. Beginning that same year, in order to overcome the problems created by sheer size, the house staff on the West Campus (Montefiore and NCB) was divided into three medical services, each with its own director and chief resident. The interns were responsible for the daily care and supervision of all patients under the guidance of more experienced residents and attending physicians. House officers wrote all orders and were responsible for the initial work-up and evaluation of all patients as well as some laboratory tests. Routine laboratory work was done by the hospital labs, and morning blood samples were drawn by a special phlebotomy team. Interns spent time at Montefiore and North Central Bronx while some also went to White Plains Hospital, a suburban hospital with which an affiliation had been recently established. On the East Campus house staff rotated through Bronx Municipal Hospital Center and the College Hospital.

James Scheuer, M.D., the vice-chairman of the department in charge of the program at Montefiore, was Director of the Division of Cardiology, with wide-ranging research activities in clinical electrophysiology, nuclear cardiology, clinical pharmacology, and ventricular function, as well as pacemakers and cardiac physiology and metabolism.

During the negotiations with the College over the shape of the Unified Department of Medicine, the old disagreement over whether there should be a separate Department of Oncology surfaced. Edward Greenwald, Acting Chairman of Oncology, was a second-generation physician at Montefiore, following in the footsteps of his mother. In 1979, he wrote about the progress made in cancer treatment: "Uterine choriocarcinoma, formerly universally fatal, now rarely leads to death. Radiotherapy and/or chemotherapy have enabled us to cure as many as 75 percent of patients with Hodgkin's disease below the age of fifty."

The debate about the viability of a separate department was settled with the appointment of Dr. Peter Wiernik as Gutman Professor and Chairman of the Department of Oncology at Montefiore and Director of the Medical Oncology Division of the Department of Medicine at the College. Coming from the Baltimore Cancer Research Center, he was as optimistic as Greenwald about the future: "In the last decade cancer has proven to be one of the diseases most amenable to medical, surgical, and radiotherapeutic intervention."

Irwin Merkatz came from the Midwest to chair the combined Department of Obstetrics and Gynecology. Robert Ruben accepted the chairmanship of unified Otolaryngology; Selwyn Freed, Urology; Robert Katzman, Neurology; and M. Donald Blaufox, Nuclear Medicine.

In the late seventies, another change in power relationships occurred. As long as Montefiore was a hospital specializing in the care of the chronically ill, covering the entire metropolitan area, a Board of Trustees drawn from a particular group of well-to-do philanthropists seemed appropriate. As the Hospital became an institution serving the immediate Bronx community for all health-care needs, Cherkasky felt the need to involve the people who used the Hospital in the decisions that were made. The first vehicles for participation were the advisory boards set up for various neighborhood clinics, culminating in a Community Advisory Board watching over the whole Hospital. When three members from that board and one from the community at large were elected to the Board of Trustees, now under the leadership of Robert Tishman, a powerful force in real estate in New York City, Montefiore became the first voluntary hospital in the city to share ultimate legal authority with representatives of the community served by the Hospital. The Auxiliary continued its earlier role of devising innovative services to patients, especially of education and advocacy.

Some of the power struggles typical of American medicine were played out at Montefiore in a highly idiosyncratic form. The "full-time principle" of physicians on salary was originally advocated to improve the quality of teaching at medical schools. Bluestone wanted to put doctors on salary at Montefiore because he disapproved of fee-for-service medicine, feeling that piecework, an income dependent on seeing more and more patients, doing more and more procedures, was not a good way to practice medicine, the corollary being that medical care should be available to those who needed it, not just those who could pay for it. He put his chiefs and other physicians on salary; Home Care and Medical Group were staffed by physicians on salary. Cherkasky agreed. Their programs happened to fit the peculiar condition of Jewish physicians and hospitals in New York City of the period and, over the years, became attractive to department chiefs and others with quite different agendas, concerned with objectives originally important to the improvement of academic medicine. For fifty years, from the arrival of Lichtwitz in the early thirties, Montefiore had a higher proportion of physicians on salary than any other voluntary hospital. By 1961, there were 64 physicians on full-time salary; by 1971, 463 on salary (256 full-time and 207 part-time); by 1981, 573 (315 full-time, 258 part-time). They had been added to staff the outreach programs and to strengthen teaching, research, and patient care.

The voluntary physicians saw the development as a threat, believing that the salaried staff had easier access to Hospital resources, to beds for their patients, to operating room time, while they brought their patients and thus income to the institution, did much of the teaching, and thought of themselves as role models for the residents-in-training. Medical Board meetings were frequently scenes of complaint about difficulties in obtaining beds for admission and accusations that programs like the neighborhood health centers created demands for beds and treatment that the Hospital could not meet.

By the time of Cherkasky's approaching retirement the picture was changing. The attempts of the federal and state governments to control rising health-care costs made the support of such a large full-time staff difficult. Many of the salaried physicians had always treated private patients, their contracts specifying how much of the income they generated was theirs to keep, how much went back to the Hospital or the department for the support of research. As funds were cut or lagged behind inflation, salaried physicians found themselves under pressure to earn more from private practice. Those who had chosen salaries because they did not like the demands of private practice found this unpalatable. The voluntary physicians saw this as further evidence of institutional prejudice and competition directed at them. The situation was increasingly exacerbated by physical overcrowding.

CHAPTER

18

Transition

As he approached retirement Cherkasky was a slight man of middle height with a bright mane of white hair. People who heard tales of his room-dominating personality were sometimes surprised on meeting him until they sensed the force of obsessive energy. He never appeared relaxed. Sitting at his desk reading or signing papers, he was wholly focused on the task. In the hospital halls, he either walked head thrust forward in concentration, recognizing no one around him, or stopped to greet colleague, patient, or employee with an equal mixture of charm and concern, seeming never to forget a face, a name, the details of an illness, a hobby, an interest, or the worries about a favorite child. The regard for people was real, but also part of his managerial style and a reason for administrative effectiveness. The secretary whose husband was a total invalid was tied by bonds of hopeless loyalty to the employer who expressed such profound and caring sympathy.

The physical image he projected was more that of anguished saint or Miltonic Satan than that of politician. There was always an air of physical fragility about him and this increased with age, as if the nonessentials had dropped away and the intense personality burned through the flesh. His usually tanned skin set off the white hair, the clothes meticulously fresh, small feet clad in neat black slip-on shoes.

The imagery of saintliness was suggested, not by any emanations of simple moral goodness, but by the sense that here was someone who had his eyes fixed on a grail that others would not or could not see. He seemed forever engaged in a quest that was larger than life, and was capable often of persuading others in a room to catch a momentary glimpse of something that made them feel that they too were working in an undertaking of moment.

A presentation of the year's budget to the Distribution Committee of the Federation of Jewish Philanthropies became high drama. The committee, sitting through a week of budgets from Federation agencies, hospitals, community centers, day camps, all worthy, none even slightly different from the year before, had reached a level of profound torpor when Cherkasky and his staff arrived. Assistants laid out budgets for Montefiore and an affiliated facility with no noticeable change in the waters. Cherkasky spoke and not only created ripples but transformed the pond to a lake and then to a wide ocean. He talked about negotiations with the union, and this became a matter for the upcoming state elections. He talked about Montefiore's desire to preserve the surrounding neighborhood from the creeping destruction of the South Bronx, and this became a discussion of the fate of America's cities. He talked about the latest quarrel with the Albert Einstein College of Medicine, and this was not a minor academic brawl, but a tragedy that could result in a "great loss to the worldwide Jewish community." A dull afternoon of the civilities of professional philanthropy was lifted to a level of high seriousness, and a group of bored officials was reminded that there was an ultimate purpose of some dignity to their deliberations.

Cherkasky did not succeed in rationalizing the hospital system of New York City. The prediction he made in 1968 that "the time is coming when everybody in the country will have comprehensive health insurance coverage" was not fulfilled. In general, medical education had not changed very much, even in the college with which he was most closely associated. The dichotomy of purpose within Montefiore still ran deep.

On occasion, he regretted aloud the compromises made in the process of building Montefiore's reputation as a first-class hospital judged by the standards of the medical establishment: "The price of that commitment is that we are, with some notable exceptions, not so different from other institutions. I have all kinds of people who could just as easily be transported to the labs or halls of hospitals (of which there are many) which don't really care much about things that we claim we care about. It's been a failure, a real failure."

Few observers—either enemies or friends—agreed with that assessment. He showed that change was possible, that, through careful planning, practical examples of reform could be created inside and outside Montefiore. City hospitals were in measurably better shape than when he first made his reports. Far more people in the United States had access to medical care than thirty years before—and he had played an important role in that extension. During his lifetime, the American medical system never lacked for critics. Blueprints for improvement constantly rolled from the presses. The articles that Cherkasky published over the years were interesting in that context. Few were purely theoretical. Almost all described programs implemented by Montefiore: Home Care, the Medical Group, the Family Health Maintenance Demonstration, the Mosholu-Montefiore Community Center, the Loeb Center, the Martin Luther King, Jr., Health Care Center, and so on down through the years. He was no tilter against windmills. He was the constructive critic, creating models, putting his own and other people's ideas into concrete form, showing how the existing resources could be used to design new and different ways of delivering health care, how that seemingly immovable system could be manipulated and pulled into a more useful shape, building prototypes that others might replicate or modify for their own circumstances.

He chose to fight his battles for better medical care at the heart of the system. While some of the innovative programs functioned at a physical distance from the Hospital, they were closely integrated with Montefiore's training and research tracks. The medical school curriculum might be untouched, but residents spending time at an ambulatory-care center had experiences quite different from those at the familiar bedside. The team philosophy and practical democracy of a residency in social medicine produced a physician with different skills from those developed in a more traditional setting. Some people came to learn and work at Montefiore because they were attracted by the radical reputation of Cherkasky and his hospital. Others found themselves changed by the experience of being there.

Constant vigilance was part of the price paid to preserve the less traditional departments against encroachment and attack, to make sure that the graduates of the more innovative programs were accepted on a level of equality, and to find the resources to make sure that all the divergent forces were healthily sustained.

He was to protect and preserve some of his most precious experiments over many years. Above all, he was able to sustain his own enthusiasm for the fray, his sense of values, his awareness of the world around, and his instinct for teaching others how to implement ideals in a less than perfect world.

On a cold January night in 1981, thirty years after he had taken over the leadership of Montefiore and a few months from retirement, Cherkasky met with his Board of Trustees and spent the evening teaching them about the problems of the Hospital within the context of the current state of the community and the city. He talked about the difficulties of recruiting a top-flight chairman for the combined Department of Obstetrics-Gynecology in a complex where most of the obstetrical beds were in municipal hospitals suffering severely from the cutbacks in funding from New York City. He went on to talk about the effects of the same diminution of city money on other areas in the same hospitals functioning as sections of combined departments, warning the Board that city cutbacks were creating a critical drain on Montefiore resources.

Now he wanted the Board of Trustees to become involved in supporting and strengthening the community that still existed around the Hospital, persuading them to lend their time and money and talents to the cause. The prelude to the meeting had been months of conversation with staff, with individual Board members, with committees. The immediate sequel was more talk, more persuasion, as Cherkasky walked through the halls of the Hospital with two Trustees, inviting them to ride downtown with him, continuing their education, explaining the possibilities, catching them up in his own enthusiasm, enlisting them in his endless quest.

He left the institution facing two immediate problems. Plans had not yet been approved for the desperately needed construction program. Eleven years had been occupied by the long process of seeking approval at all separate levels.

The institution was also left with a very small endowment fund. Cherkasky's drive for independence from his Board of Trustees led him to concentrate on raising money from government or foundation grants. Neither allowed for the accumulation of money in the bank or a sufficient contingency fund. The plans for construction as finally approved called for an expenditure of around $250 million. Ten percent of that had to be raised as a down payment on the mortgage.

The new Chairman of the Board was Lawrence Buttenwieser, related to many of the members through a family at the center of New York's German Jewish aristocracy. Much of his energy was to be used in efforts to raise the money, a difficult feat with a Board that had not been asked for large sums of money for many years and an institution that had not asked either the public or its physicians for donations over an equally long period of time.

The Board provided continuity. Membership changed slowly. There were around fifty members, the term of office usually ending only with death. Younger members learned under the tutelage of the experienced. The collective memory was long. Ex-Presidents Tishman and Rosenthal continued to serve, actively involved with the medical, social and financial problems of the eighties.

Buttenwieser presided over a Board of Trustees which, in some essentials, was similar to that which had presided over the twenty-six beds in the original Home for Chronic Invalids. Ultimate legal responsibility for the operation of the modern Medical Center still lay with the Trustees: a heavy financial responsibility in these days of expensive medicine, public mistrust of physicians and hospitals, and the threat of bankruptcy hovering over many of the hospitals most devoted to the public good. Most members of the Board were still important figures in the New York world of law, finance, and real estate, the skills learned in their business lives the skills brought to discussions at Board meetings. Many of them were descendants of the original members of the Board and they brought to their deliberations the same mixture of concerns about individual patients, general social conditions, and the direction of the institution which had motivated their great-grandfathers.

There were two groups on the Board quite different from the men who had played poker with Jacob Schiff on Sunday mornings. Since 1928, there had been women on the Board. They were frequently also members of the Auxiliary and through their work in that organization had a perspective on the life of the Medical Center from a viewpoint unlike that of most of the men. Few of the male members of the Board could now spend very much time at Montefiore. Distance was a problem, as it had been since the move to the North Bronx. Many members of the Auxiliary, however, spent long days at the Medical Center: they sat in the booth outside the operating suite, giving information and comfort to waiting families; they sat behind the tables of the Information and Referral Service, helping bewildered patients find their way through the maze of welfare and other desperately needed services; they provided help and companionship to mothers and children waiting in the clinics; working behind the counters of the gift shop, they listened to the concerns and complaints of visitors and staff. Using their funds as seed money for pioneering programs, they learned at first hand about the life of the Bronx. They brought this knowledge back to Board deliberations.

The other new group consisted of the numbers elected by the Community Advisory Board. These were people who lived and worked in the Bronx, aware, through personal experience, of the hazards faced by the young and the old, the dangers of the streets and the difficulties of their constituents in finding their way into an increasingly complex and bureaucratic health care system.

Thus, while the Board members were no longer able to talk with each patient or read each application for admission, many were still in close touch with the daily life of the Center. Buttenwieser encouraged close contact on the part of the others: urging them to donate blood, to visit as much as possible, insisting that patient food be served at Board meetings, as eager for their involvement as had been Jacob Schiff when Trustees, obeying his injunction, waited on street corners for him to pick them up and drive them to meetings.

This was a Board which followed traditions of sound financial management, linked with the ability to empathize with the pain of others. A discussion about the ramifications of a restructuring of the Board which aroused all the hair-splitting instincts to argument of the lawyers' minds around the table was followed by a physician's presentation of the legal and moral dilemmas created by that newly won expertise in saving the lives of premature babies. This was also a discussion of the law, but concerns of the heart were more apparent as the Trustees considered the fates of these, the smallest of their charges. Another physician and an administrator described the work of the hospice program, designed to care for the dying. Time seemed to have stood still for a hundred years. Then the patients applying for admission had needed a doctor's assurance that they were incurable. Applicants to the hospice program were the terminally ill, expected to die within six months. The physician told of the last weeks of a young woman dying of cancer and brought from her own uncomfortable, difficult home to a hospice room, where the first concerns of staff were to comfort her and relieve her pain. Her fate and the help offered at Montefiore were little different from the stories of those first young women who had come to the Home for Chronic Invalids with blood-soaked lungs or inoperable tumors. The physician told of another patient, a recent immigrant from Russia, who knew that he was leaving his elderly wife frightened and alone in a strange land. The Board members listened as they had listened to similar stories for a hundred years. They listened and offered support for the programs that provided more than medical care as the answer to pain.

Much of the Board's time had always been concerned, not with these directly human affairs, but with matters of finance and planning. Now they were equally concerned with government regulation. When Henry Moses wished to improve the hospital, he was able to take direct action, to generously donate the money for a betatron. The latest in modern technology, CAT scanners were regulated by government fiat. Permission had to be sought for the purchase.

The Trustees were free to follow Moses' leadership in other directions: to use their skills as lawyers and businessmen to guide the institution through the problems of planning and financing new programs, to keep as closely abreast of the constant new discoveries of medical science as was possible for intelligent lay citizens, to develop a close working relationship with the administrative staff, to listen to the voices of all the groups at Montefiore—the physicians, the nurses, the administrators, the workers, the patients.

Continuity was also provided by physicians who remained, after formal retirement, active participants in the life of the Medical Center. Louis Leiter continued to advise younger colleagues. Harry Zimmerman, who had done so much to build both the Medical Center and the College of Medicine, whose international reputation in pathology continued to reflect glory on Montefiore, was still bouncingly active, talking with Board members and professional colleagues about appointments to the staff, about fund raising, about plans for the coming hundredth birthday celebration.

The man chosen by the Board to take the helm in the summer of 1981 was from an academic background, and when Carl Eisdorfer became President of Montefiore, he was also appointed a professor in the Departments of Psychiatry and Neuroscience at the Albert Einstein College of Medicine. Born in New York

City, he received his Bachelor's, Master's and Ph.D. degrees from New York University and an M.D. from Duke University School of Medicine, where he spent sixteen years as a member of the faculty and directed the medical school's Behavioral Sciences Program as well as the Duke University Center for the Study of Aging and Human Development. He then went to the University of Washington in Seattle to become chairman of the Department of Psychiatry and Behavioral Science at the School of Medicine. He was Founding Director of the university's Institute on Aging, his major scientific and clinical research concentrated in the fields of gerontology, psychology, and psychiatry. A member of the Institute of Medicine of the National Academy of Sciences, he spent a sabbatical year in 1980 as Senior Scholar in Residence at the Institute of Medicine. He worked actively on policy and programs for the elderly, serving on the Federal Council on Aging and the National Advisory Council of the National Institute on Aging. He saw the increasing number of people surviving to old age as one of the major challenges facing the United States. In 1900, aged Americans comprised 3.1 percent of the population; by 1980, this increased to approximately 11 percent of the population (23 million people), the number expected to exceed 31 million—about 13 to 15 percent of the population—by the turn of the century and to grow to a substantial 18 to 29 percent by the year 2020.

Eisdorfer, a psychiatrist with a special interest in the problems of aging, took over an institution with a high proportion of elderly patients. Indeed, the Moses Division cared for more Medicare patients than any other major institution in the country. The Bronx had a large proportion of two kinds of people, the very young and the very old, and the old were getting older. Physicians began to refer to the "young-old" and the "old-old." By 1983, there were 18,000 people over the age of eighty-five in the borough, and calculations were made that by the next year, half the aged population of the Bronx would be seventy-five or over.

The elderly were the concern of many different sections of the unified departments of Medicine, Neurology, and Surgery; all worked with the Resnick Gerontology Center at the College to develop programs for the elderly. The Medical Group, still serving many of the original enrollees, found more than 100 patients between seventy-five and eighty-five years of age to participate in a Bronx Aging Study. The volunteers received yearly physical examinations, neuropsychological testing, and twenty-four-hour electrocardiograms at yearly intervals for five years, the purpose to determine parameters of normal physical and mental health for people of this age.

The Division of Geriatrics, under David Hamerman, former Chief of Medicine, began interdisciplinary Geriatric Rounds. Certain selected elderly patients benefited from an intervention program in which specialists in geriatric medicine, neurology, psychiatry, and rehabilitation medicine, together with a pharmacist, social worker, geriatric nurse-practitioner, home nurse coordinator, nutritionist, and lawyer, assessed their mental states and ability to function. Together the professionals developed a comprehensive health-care plan for these patients designed to help them return home whenever possible.

Some patients, after their acute illnesses were stabilized, were referred to a Geriatric Nursing Unit, where nurse and patient worked together to restore as much functional capacity as possible before discharge. Many elderly patients went to the Loeb Center for Nursing and Rehabilitation. Genrose Alfano, the Director, received a grant from the Robert Wood Johnson Foundation to allow her staff to follow some patients into their homes, reinforcing the methods they had been taught for their own care and keeping a continuous check on their progress. These patients were to be compared with a control group who did not have this kind of follow-up care.

The Department of Psychiatry had a Division of Aging and Geriatric Psychiatry. Its Geriatric Family Diagnostic and Treatment Service offered evaluation and care for Alzheimer's disease, depression, and other problems of the elderly, all with a strong emphasis on support for families coping with their older members. The Robert Wood Johnson Foundation allocated $6.5 million to a Program for Hospital Initiatives in Long-Term Care to guide and support the efforts of ten hospitals, over a four-year period, to develop imaginative approaches to comprehensive health care for the elderly, with Eisdorfer as director of the program and senior program consultant to the Foundation. Montefiore also expressed its institutional interest in the elderly through affiliation with the Nathan Miller Nursing Homes, one voluntary, one proprietary, in White Plains.

There were those who pointed out that this population group was, of necessity, going to disappear and that there was not an equal number of the middle-aged in the area to replace them. Statisticians suggested that planning for the future should concentrate on the large numbers of young adults and their small children who were moving into the area. Others were distressed because they did not think that the elderly were a separate category or should be treated as such. Many physicians felt that these were the same patients that they had treated for years and that they could provide more effective continuing care than some newly arrived specialist.

The Montefiore Medical Center now had an annual operating budget of around $250,000,000 and was as much a changing entity as ever. Montefiore Hospital, renamed the Henry and Lucy Moses Division in honor of the couple who had given so much to the institution over the years, had 890 beds, including Loeb. Next door, connected by bridges and a city contract, was North Central Bronx, with 398 beds. On another corner of the acreage once filled with lawns and trees was the Mosholu-Montefiore Community Center, still providing services to patients and employees. Ten minutes away by car was the Beth Abraham Hospital with 504 beds for long-term care, linked to Montefiore by board memberships. In 1983, a fifty-year lease was signed for the operation of the Hospital of the Albert Einstein College of Medicine with its 431 beds. The Moses Division, NCB, and HAECOM among them accommodated around half a million outpatient and emergency visits a year. The Martin Luther King, Jr., Health Center had become an independent body in the late seventies, but Montefiore still provided ambulatory care for the prisoners at Rikers Island, for families in the Bronx at the Comprehensive Health

Care Center, which had 29,046 patients enrolled, and at the Family Health Center, which served 9,724 people, and for 3,475 families in Yonkers at the Valentine Lane Family Practice.

The more than 1,500 physicians who worked in all these places dealt with the entire spectrum of disease and disability. None of the problems that had afflicted the original Montefiore patients had disappeared: tuberculosis was no longer an epidemic but had never been eliminated from the slums of the Bronx; drug addiction was probably more prevalent than in the nineteenth century; arthritis and neurological diseases such as multiple sclerosis were still cripplers; the death rate from heart disease and stroke was dropping but the treatment of these conditions probably absorbed more time and resources than any other throughout the complex; cancer patients were no longer doomed to a quick death, treatment steadily becoming more effective; syphilis and the other venereal diseases were still endemic, although treatable.

In the late 1970s and early 1980s infectious diseases reappeared as a widespread threat with a terrifying effect on the public psyche. First there was Legionnaire's disease, named from the American Legion convention at which it first came to notice; then toxic shock syndrome. Genital herpes spread as a national epidemic. Dr. Ilya Spigland, head of the Division of Virology, tried to stem the panic: "Everybody has some form of herpes. Everyone who has ever had chicken pox carries the virus. Genital herpes is simply a variation of a very common disorder. Some people have one outbreak of lesions and never have another. Other people have recurrent outbreaks, although I believe they would have far fewer recurrences if they stopped being obsessed by it." Then in 1981, AIDS, acquired immune deficiency syndrome, surfaced. Within two years the problem was recognized in thirty-five states and the District of Columbia in 1,450 cases, causing 558 known deaths. Half of the cases occurred in New York City. AIDS appeared to show up chiefly in four high-risk groups: homosexual and bisexual men, people taking drugs intravenously, Haitian immigrants, and hemophiliacs dependent on blood transfusions. Women who showed symptoms were thought to have had sexual contact with infected men. When the syndrome began to show up in babies born at the Hospital of Albert Einstein College of Medicine, Dr. Neal Steigbigel, who headed the Division of Infectious Diseases, warned that AIDS "would, therefore, have to be considered a potential threat to the general population. Just how much of a threat is unknown."

No one knew the cause, whether it was a totally new agent or an old one acting in a new way. Its effect was to destroy the body's immune system, leaving the victim open to any kind of infection. The distinctive characteristics were fever, weight loss, extreme fatigue, lymph node enlargement, and a rare cancer, Kaposi's sarcoma.

Each outbreak of infectious disease engendered a certain public hysteria in a nation that had come to believe that the specter of dangerous infections had been laid to rest by antibiotics and vaccines. While trying to calm unnecessary fears, Spigland worked on monitoring pregnant women in danger of passing along their own herpes infection to their unborn children, recommending a cesarean section if there was a flare-up of infection close to the expected date of birth. He was also investigating the role of an organism called chlamydia in genital infections, suspecting that it was a much more important agent than had previously been suspected.

Answers to several of the compelling medical questions of the eighties—the resurgence of the threat of infectious diseases, the problem of transplant rejection, and the riddle of why some people develop cancer and others, apparently equally at risk, do not—seemed to lie within the body's immune system. This was the area where Parviz Lalezari, head of the Division of Immunohematology, worked. Apart from developing new techniques for sorting and storing varieties of blood, his basic interest was in antibody-antigen reaction, his research in autoimmune diseases, diseases in which the body attacks itself. He had begun to look at people at the level of individual tissues, to classify the antigens and eventually to match kidney for kidney, pancreas for pancreas, skin for skin, and so on.

The immediate problem was the physical plant in which these investigations took place. Eleven years after the first application, preliminary permission to begin a $250 million construction program arrived, leaving the continuing severe problems of overcrowding until building could be completed.

The Moses Division was the scene of constant conflict over the overcrowded operating rooms. Only one had been added to the ten built in the early fifties. Not only had the number of procedures increased greatly; they had increased enormously in complexity and the length of time required. A bypass operation took four or five hours; reimplantation of a limb, fifteen or sixteen hours. The aftercare required by patients undergoing these complicated operations was longer and more dependent on machines, which also took up space. The operating rooms were a traffic jam; the recovery rooms, designed for the simpler days of years before, a bottleneck. Almost every medical staff meeting brought bitter complaints about the situation from frustrated surgeons, or reports from hopeful administrators who thought they had found a new way of cutting up the pie. After two years of negotiation with New York City, Montefiore was able to lease one of the operating rooms at North Central Bronx.

The emergency room was as critically short of space as the operating room area. As a hospital for chronic diseases, Montefiore had not needed an emergency room except to handle the odd accident to staff or patient. With the change to an acute-care institution in the fifties, emergency services were offered to the general community, and there was a brisk business in scraped knees and injuries from falls. During the next twenty years, there were great changes in the way in which emergency rooms all over the city were used, as they substituted for the family doctor or the crowded clinic. At the same time, as traffic, violence, and fires increased in the Bronx, cases of trauma grew. As demands for beds proliferated, patients coming into the Hospital through the emergency room could not be admitted quickly enough.

The emergency rooms at Montefiore and North Central Bronx

took care of ten times as many patients each year as Montefiore alone had cared for twenty years before.

Patients moved in and out of beds in the Hospital much more quickly. In the same twenty years, the average length of stay had decreased from 45 days to 10.5 days. These patients were, however, much sicker. The care they received was much more concentrated. In 1962, 12,031 patients were admitted to beds at Montefiore Hospital; in 1982, the equivalent figure (admissions to the Henry and Lucy Moses Division) was 25,540. The number of laboratory procedures had leaped from around half a million to over five million. Patients spent their time in the Hospital undergoing active medical care: tests, X-rays, surgery. For recuperation they went home, to the Loeb Center, to Beth Abraham, or to nursing homes. A striking indication of how sick these patients were is that although the number of patients admitted each year more than doubled, the number of meals served in a year actually decreased, from 1,094,190 to 1,031,574. These patients were too sick to eat.

Halting decay in the neighborhood was another priority. The Mosholu Preservation Corporation was set up with a board composed of Montefiore Trustees and community representatives, with a paid director. This independent corporation took two pathways. In the first year it bought and renovated two apartment buildings and negotiated acquisition and mortgage financing of two others, adding up to 315 apartments. Becoming a major landlord or creating a cordon sanitaire around the Medical Center was not the basic aim of the Corporation. Much of the staff's time and energy went into serving as technical adviser to owners of neighborhood apartment buildings who wanted to improve their properties, keeping them informed of refinancing and rehabilitation programs, helping them to prepare applications, and participating on their behalf in negotiations with private lenders and public officials.

Ethnic diversity marked the ownership and merchandise of the small stores that survived under the El on Jerome Avenue, up and down the steep slopes of Gun Hill Road and the gentle fall of Bainbridge Avenue. There were delicatessens with pastrami and knishes and bagels and lox; there was the Emergency Cuban Restaurant, which served "coffee express and Cuban sandwiches"; there were restaurants that served "Chinas Comidas" and an Indian lunch counter with pakooras and chapatis.

In the neighborhood, the economic impact of the people who worked at Montefiore was considerable: they ate lunch at the local restaurants and shopped on Jerome Avenue. There was also institutional recognition that the small shopkeepers contributed to the stability of the neighborhood. The Mosholu Preservation Corporation and the Jerome Avenue Merchants Association together developed a privately funded program to provide electronic burglary, fire, and robbery surveillance of the local stores by a computerized system at the Hospital.

Trustees and members of the Auxiliary took a part in setting up another independent corporation designed to help the neighborhood. Bronx Community Enterprises aimed to nurture commercial and industrial development in the area by encouraging new businesses that would bring in jobs and income. Where possible, the purchasing power of the Medical Center was used to help the fledgling operations.

A new group of poverty-stricken immigrants with desperate problems arrived, unheralded and unnoticed until the members of the staff of the Family Health Center on 193rd Street saw a small child playing naked in the street. He proved to be one of about 700 Cambodian refugees brought to the North Bronx by resettlement agencies from refugee camps in Thailand. The agencies neglected to alert local services or community groups to the arrival of the Cambodians, who were living, mostly without jobs, resources, or the ability to speak much English, in unheated and shabby apartments.

Once the first contact was made—a diaper for the child— scores of Cambodians quickly found their way to the Center, asking for help with everything from medical problems to utility bills. When the staff in turn visited the Cambodians at home, they found deplorable living conditions: sewage seeping into some rooms, no electricity, vermin. Many had spent their first winter in a cold climate without warm clothes or blankets. Many had severe health problems, such as parasites or tuberculosis. The children were rapidly acquiring the scourge of the Bronx, high levels of lead in their bodies. (They may have been particularly susceptible because of poor nutrition.)

Their life stories were pathetic. One woman who had two living children reported that she had given birth eight times. The other babies had all died of starvation. These were mainly rural people trying to adjust to a totally foreign environment.

Robert Massad, the Chairman of Family Medicine, and Jack O'Connor, head of Community Affairs, worked with government agencies and community groups to find the money and resources to help. They were able to hire a Cambodian interpreter, herself a refugee, who translated not only the patients' language but also their customs and attitudes. Local organizations and individuals helped. A mailman spread the news of a clothing drive.

Montefiore prepared to celebrate its one hundredth birthday surrounded by difficulties, both certain and uncertain. Construction of the new buildings was begun and the manifold problems of attempting to carry on the day-to-day business of a hospital while demolishing and rebuilding were painfully obvious. The long years of delay during a period of rapid inflation of the dollar meant that the construction when complete would probably be immediately inadequate. The Bronx was still a symbol of urban decay. The special squad set up by the city of New York to fight fires in the most arson-prone areas moved into the North Bronx.

Administrators who worried about the increasing numbers of Medicaid patients or those with no coverage who came to Montefiore looked north to Westchester County and beyond for patients less threatening to the financial stability of the institution.

The health care system was in a period of great uncertainty: the for-profit chains draining off funds and in many localities altering the structure of care; the surplus of physicians growing. For many years, the federal government had gradually cut back on support for basic scientific research and new programs for the delivery of health care.

Planning was always a difficult exercise in medicine. Administrators, Trustees, and physicians alike, deciding upon future teaching programs or purchases of equipment, pondered the question of whether cardiac surgery would continue to grow or whether other solutions would be found for the ills of the heart. So much money and so much in the way of human resources had been devoted to cancer and, while methods of treatment constantly improved, there was still no clear direction toward the ultimate answer, whether prevention or cure. The number of transplants continued to grow, with some organs appearing much more amenable to human manipulation than others, as new drugs helped overcome the problem of rejection. Infection still stalked hospital wards and broke out in the community in novel and threatening forms often enough to be a recurring reality.

There were still no answers to some of the diseases from which the original patients had suffered: arthritis, the scleroses, and other neurological conditions. Poverty had certainly not been eliminated from New York as a contributing factor to ill health.

On the other hand, there were some achievements. Collaboration with the Albert Einstein College of Medicine was a reality on many levels. Together the two institutions made up one of the largest and most respected medical complexes in the country, assured of national and international recognition in many fields, providing the most complex tertiary care to patients who came from all over the world and from the next street.

At the same time, Montefiore remained true to the vision of Jacob Schiff and Simon Baruch. Whether named a "Home" or a "Hospital" or a "Medical Center," this was an institution where missions were interpreted broadly; where taking care of the family of the immigrant tailor was as important as taking care of his lungs; where doctors thought it was important to go out into the slums and the prisons in search of patients. The founding fathers would have agreed with Cherkasky when he said:

"Throughout its history, Montefiore has always been both on the leading edge of science and at the center of human service, striving to care for the patient with warmth and compassion and parceling out its resources in such a way that we further the bright hopes scientific medicine holds for the future while meeting all the needs of those, inside and outside our walls, who look to us for succor."

Notes on Sources

The problem with the records of a modern medical center is quantity: memos, computer printouts, reports to accreditation, reimbursement, and regulatory agencies, minutes, bills, legal documents, and the endless stream of paper generated by a profession in which peer recognition and advancement are alike dependent upon publication. The researcher turns with relief to the relative paucity of nineteenth-century records.

Montefiore has been particularly fortunate that, although until recently no consistent efforts were made to save or store the old records, a large amount survived, not complete, but enough to allow for an understanding of much that happened in the early days. They include:

Patient Records

These are on microfilm and computer from 1917 on. The records from before that date are in the same volumes into which the handwritten loose pages were originally bound. Not all of these volumes have been found, but there are enough to indicate the general trends in medical care and the specific treatments of hundreds of patients, with considerable material on their background and behavior while in the Home for Chronic Invalids.

Minutes of the Board of Trustees and Its Executive Committee

From 1884 until after the turn of the century, these were handwritten into large books. Since the Trustees were frequent visitors to and active participants in the day-to-day business of the Home, the minutes contain much detailed information about routine matters. From around 1908 (by which time the typewriter had succeeded the pen), only scattered remnants of these minutes have been found until the record again becomes more or less complete from about 1940 to the present day.

Annual Reports

From 1884 to 1934, when the Depression curtailed production, these appeared every year. After that, they appeared only intermittently. These later reports were all produced by public relations departments and each reflected only one point of view, that of the administrator of the Board of Trustees. Those of the first fifty years, on the other hand, contained not only the accounts of the Board of Trustees but independently written reports by various physicians and heads of departments, often presenting divergent opinions.

Minutes of the Medical Board

A small book contains these minutes dating from 1893 to 1918, expressing the concerns of the physicians and providing a running account of the organization of a professional staff.

The Montefiore Echo

This four-page news bulletin was printed free by a local business. From 1915 until 1928 it was written and edited by the patients. When Bluestone came as Director in 1928, he took over the *Echo* as an official publication and the patients' point of view disappeared from its pages.

Autopsy Reports

In an institution that valued the autopsy so highly, the reports were treasured. From 1913 they were bound in annual volumes and they provide not only a method of checking diagnosis but considerable information about the state of medical science at any given time.

Professional Papers

With its tradition of social concern, Montefiore has been the source of a vast literature on the organization of medicine and other health-related issues produced by both physicians and administrators.

From 1917 on, copies of papers published in scientific journals by staff members were bound in annual volumes. The practice began with Boas and the first volume covers the years 1917 to 1922. One has appeared each year since then except for the World War II years. While obviously all the papers are available from other sources, the year-by-year collection offers an overview of institutional directions.

Photographs

Pride in the new building produced a series of photographs of interiors in 1889 to begin a collection that now covers almost one hundred years and often provides information not available in the written record.

Interviews

I have had the opportunity to interview many Montefiore people, most of whom consented to the use of a tape recorder, so that there is now in existence a large library of interviews with physicians, administrators, social workers, nurses, patients, and so on, beginning chronologically with a man who started to work at Montefiore while the institution was still in Manhattan and helped with the move to the Bronx in 1913.

Newspapers

Nineteenth-century coverage of Montefiore in both the Jewish and the general press focused on social news: the Fair of 1886, the charitable activities of well-to-do businessmen and their wives and daughters. After the stories about the introduction of insulin in 1923, the Hospital was viewed more and more as a source of scientific news.

Unpublished Papers and Theses

Over the years, many students, either visitors or staff, wrote papers about Montefiore programs and procedures in fulfillment of degree requirements of various institutions. These often had as their subjects the experimental or the innovative.

Other Materials

Information lies in many accidentally preserved sources: programs from special events such as ground breakings and dinners; pamphlets distributed to incoming patients with lists of rules to be followed; the "Precedent Books" with rules for interns, residents, and nurses; diet manuals; a scrapbook put together by the daughter of one of the first Trustees containing invitations, newspaper clippings, minutes of meetings, etc.; the minutes of the Staff and Alumni Association.

Index

Index

Botstein, Charles, 223, 227
brain surgery, 182
Brandeis University, 246
breast cancer, 99–100
Bright's disease, 26, 89
bromides, 59
bronchitis, 30, 71
Bronx, South, *see* South Bronx
Bronx Community Abortion Center, 276
Bronx Community Enterprises, 315
Bronx Municipal Hospital Center (BMHC), 224, 263, 286, 287, 291, 294, 296
Bronx Women's Liberation Group, 276
Brooklyn Federation of Jewish Charities, 105
Brooks, Harlow, 88
Bullowa, Jesse, 59
Burk, Peter, 295
Burritt, Bailey, 197
Buseck, Otto, 68
Buttenwieser, Lawrence, 304, 305, 306

caffeine and antipyrin, combination of, 60
calcium: metabolism of, 222, 295; and strontium-90, 222
Cambodian refugees in North Bronx, 316, 317
camphor, 60
Canada, 249
cancer, 98, 99, 118, 122, 136, 163, 191, 204, 205, 297, 311, 312; breast, 99–100; chemotherapy for, 296; of colon, 220; endometrial, 267; of esophagus, 221; lung, 100, 185, 213; radiotherapy for, 99, 135, 223, 297; two main types of, 99; *see also* carcinomas; sarcomas
carcinomas, 99, 100, 180, 267, 296; *see also* cancer
cardiac cart, 221–2
cardiac catheterization, 178, 215–16, 219, 290, 291
cardiac hypertrophy, 59
cardiology, 118, 120, 125, 178, 215, 216, 222, 257, 258, 289, 290, 291 296; *see also* heart disease
cardiotachometer, 143, 144

Carlebach, Rosa, 169, 190
Carnegie, Andrew, 41
CAT scanners, 152, 307
cerebral palsy, 165
cesarean section, 285, 312
chemotherapy, 296
Cherkasky, Martin, 162, 163, 164, 165, 193, 196–209 *passim*, 212, 224, 225, 227, 228, 229, 230, 232, 233, 235–45 *passim*, 252, 254, 257, 258, 259, 261, 265, 274, 280, 292, 295, 297, 298, 300–4; appearance of, 300, 301; on definition of hospital, 245, 317; and education of young physicians, 285–6; fee-for-service medicine opposed by, 209; innovative programs supported by, 302, 303; in lecture at Massachusetts General Hospital (1963), 244–5; Loeb Center for Nursing and Rehabilitation built by, 240; and Montefiore Board of Trustees, 253–4, 303, 304; and Montefiore Medical Center as acute-care general hospital and teaching institution, 203; personality of, dominating, 253, 300, 301; as President of Montefiore Hospital and Medical Center, 291
Chicago, University of, 175, 211
Child Care Health Project (New York City), 272–3
Children's Bureau, U.S., 205
Chile, 273
China, 167, 272
Chinese Medical Association, 272
chlamydia, 312
chloral, 59
chloroform, 60
cholera, 10, 48, 65, 78
chorea, Sydenham's, 126
cirrhosis of liver, 69
civil rights movement, 229
Civil War, 8, 65
Cleveland, Grover, 41
cocaine, 51, 157
cod liver oil, 32, 54, 55
Cohen, Frances, 96
Cohen, Michael, 248, 293, 294
Cohn, Adele B., 167
Cohn, Felix, 93
colitis, 192, 248
Collier's magazine, 79

[3 2 5]

epinephrine, 59
Epitome of Hydrotherapy for Physicians, Architects and Nurses, An (Baruch), 47
Escher, Doris, 178, 215, 216, 290
esophagus, cancer of, 221
ether, 60
Ettinger, Leo, 57
Evander Childs High School, 107, 168

Family Health Center, 294, 311, 315
Family Health Maintenance Demonstration, 197, 198, 205, 210, 245, 302
FBI (Federal Bureau of Investigation), 207
Federal Council on Aging, 308
Federation of Jewish Philanthropies, 105, 155, 171, 172, 198, 226, 236, 301
fee-for-service medicine, 148, 155, 199, 209, 227, 298
Felbel, Mrs. Dore, 145
Feldman, A., 159
Field, Minna, 194
Finberg, Laurence, 247, 248, 256
Fineman, Solomon, 180
Fishberg, Maurice, 97, 146, 147, 156, 185
fistula in ano, 69
Flexner, Simon, 120
fluoroscopy, 291
Focht, Elizabeth F., 181
Foldes, Francis, 247
Foner, Mo, 229
Fordham Hospital, 125, 282, 283
Forlanini, Carlo, 77
Frater, Robert W. M., 287
Free Synagogue (New York City), 81, 82
Freed, Selwyn, 254, 297
Freud, Sigmund, 51, 127, 157
Friedenson, Meyer, 159, 160
Friedman, Ephraim, 286, 287
Friedman, Leo M., 167
Froelich, Dr., 26, 27
full-time principle in medicine, 154, 155, 156, 297, 298
Furman, Seymour, 219, 220, 290

Gabel, Dr., 113
Galileo, 143

gangrene, 89, 289
Gans, Louis, 21, 24
gastroenterology, 222, 243, 248, 258, 295
Gates, Frederick Taylor, 120, 121
Gates, Mrs. Frederick Taylor, 121
general paresis, 32
general practitioners, and specialists, 241
genital herpes, 311, 312
Gerber, Irwin, 279
geriatrics, 258, 309, 310; *see also* elderly; gerontology
Germany, 7, 26, 34, 52, 53, 93, 125, 129, 155, 236; Jewish emigrants from, 13, 57, 67
gerontology, 309; *see also* elderly; geriatrics
Gliedman, Marvin, 254, 255, 256, 287, 288, 291, 295
gliomas, chemically induced, 223
goiter, 113, 123, 124, 157, 179
Goldberg, Abraham, 138, 139
Goldberger, Joseph, 224
Goldman, Martin, 222
Goldsmith, Alfred N., 144
Goldstein, M. W., 121
Goldwater, S. S., 89, 93, 149
Goldwater Memorial Hospital, 172
gonorrheal perihepatitis, 294
Goodfriend, Jacob, 90, 94-5, 96
Goodhart, Simon Philip, 128
Gordon, Harry, 265
Gottlieb, Eugene, 221
Gottsegen, Irving, 211
gout, 48
Grace, William R., 41
Grand, Milton, 213
Grant, Ulysses S., 20
Grave's disease, 157
Grayzel, Arthur, 295
Grayzel, David, 236
Great Britain, 14, 34, 129, 167
Great Depression, 145, 149, 150, 151, 164, 166, 168
Great Society programs, 252, 262
Greater New York Fund, 192
Green House, 96, 211, 282
Greenwald, Edward, 296, 297
Gross, Harry, 125, 222
Gross National Product, and cost of health care, 268
Grossman, Jack, 177, 222

Index

Grossman, Shirley, 178, 196, 270
Guatemala, 274
Guerrero, Alberto García, 102
gynecology, 51, 297, 303

Habermann, Edward T., 287
Hadassah Medical Organization, 146, 149
Haimovici, Henry, 216
Hall, Lydia, 239, 240
Hallahan, Miss, 91, 106
Hallgarten, Julius, 43
Hallgarten Fund, 43
Hamerman, David, 255, 257, 309
Hampton, Wade, 9
Harmonie Club, 253, 280
Harpuder, Karl, 247
Harris, Dr., 97
Harris, Stanley E., 294
Harvard University, 127, 179
Hawker, Harry, 157
headache, 267
health, definition of, 210
Health, Education, and Welfare Department, U.S., 262, 271, 273
Health Insurance Plan (HIP) of Greater New York, 195, 196, 197, 198, 251, 269
Health Service, U.S., 222
heart disease, 59, 121, 136, 158–9, 160, 163, 174, 178, 185–6, 192, 204, 205, 207–8, 220, 222, 289, 311; *see also* cardiac catheterization; cardiac hypertrophy; cardiology; coronary bypass surgery; heart surgery; pacemaker
heart–lung machine, 217, 219
heart surgery, 208, 215, 216, 217, 218, 219, 241
Hebrew Benevolent Association (Camden, S.C.), 7
Hebrew Emigrant Aid Society, 36
Hebrew Free School Association, 15
Hebrew Immigrant Aid Society, 36
Hebrew Orphan Asylum, 27, 41, 45; Band of, 92, 109
Hebrew Sheltering Guardian Society, 45
Heimlich, Henry, 221
Heimlich Maneuver, 221
Hellman, Leon, 247

hematology, 222, 257, 258, 266, 295
Henkind, Paul, 266
Henry Street Settlement (New York City), 39
Herbert, Henry, 66–7, 69, 70
herpes, genital, 311, 312
Herskowitz, Antol, 216
Hexter, Maurice, 236
Heyman, David, 196
Hill, Ruth, 181
Hill–Burton Act, 204
Hirsch, Baron Maurice de, 34, 35, 36
Hitler, Adolf, 155, 166
HMOs, 269
Hochhauser, Edward, 83
Hochheimer, Emil, 27
Hodgkin's disease, 164, 296
Home Care, 160, 192, 193, 198, 199, 210, 212, 227, 236, 245, 279, 280, 281, 298, 302
Home for Aged and Infirm Hebrews, 17, 23, 32, 45
Homestead Act, 65
hormones: and dietary metabolism, 222; polypeptide, 295
Hospital Saturday and Sunday Association, 43, 104, 105
House Un-American Activities Committee, 207
Hudson, Perry B., 222
Hungary, 125, 191
Hurwitt, Elliott, 215, 216, 217, 218, 219, 221, 254
hydrogen, sulfurated, 30
hydrotherapy, 7, 10, 46, 47, 48, 49, 54, 62, 71, 113
Hyman, H. T., 151
hyoscine, 48, 59, 60
hyperalimentation, 71
hypertension, 59, 191
hyperthyroidism, 179, 180
hypervitaminosis D, 181
hypodermic injection, 136, 158
hypothermia, 217
hysteria, 126

immunohematology, 258, 295, 312
immunosuppressive drugs, 255
India, 167
infection, knowledge of causes of, 11, 78

Index

104, 105, 106; and vast increase in medical knowledge, 113; and World War I, 111, 114; *see also* Albert Einstein College of Medicine; Bedford Sanitarium; Montefiore Home for Chronic Invalids; Montefiore Hospital and Medical Center; Montefiore Hospital for Chronic Diseases; Montefiore Medical Center

Montefiore Home Care, *see* Home Care

Montefiore Home for Chronic Invalids, 3, 9, 13, 14, 17, 18, 25, 27, 38, 39, 45, 64, 65, 89-95 *passim*, 305, 306; autopsy rate at, 90; chemist, physiological, on staff of, 88, 89; dedication of, 19-20; discipline emphasized at, 25, 26; finances of, 21, 22, 42-3; first patient at, 19; junior house physician at, 49, 50; laboratories at, 89; managed by Executive Committee of Board of Trustees, 21, 22, 24, 49; Medical Board at, 87, 88, 91; as medical teaching center, 28; money-raising entertainments for, 41; and Montefiore Home Auxiliary Society, 42, 44; and Montefiore Home Flower Mission, 42; in move to Bronx, 92-5; nationalities and occupations of patients at, 29; as nonsectarian institution, 20; nurses at, 27, 50, 55, 90; Observation Ward at, 89; Occupational Therapy Department at, 44; pathologist on staff of, 88, 89; patients as workers at, 24; patients' reflexes tested at, 58; policy of, on admissions, 22-4; and rehabilitation of patients, 24, 29, 32, 47; research at, 45-62 *passim*; senior house physician at, 49-50, 90; specialists at, 51; treatments used at, 30-3, 47-8, 53-6, 59-62; 25th anniversary celebration of, 80, 81; *see also* Albert Einstein College of Medicine; Bedford Sanitarium; Montefiore Home and Hospital for Chronic Diseases; Montefiore Hospital and Medical Center; Montefiore Hospital for Chronic Diseases; Montefiore Medical Center

Montefiore Hospital and Medical Center, 203, 205, 207, 209, 216-24 *passim*, 227, 228, 232, 234, 237, 238, 241, 243, 244, 246, 249-67 *passim*, 270-83 *passim*, 285-99 *passim*, 301, 302, 303, 304, 305, 307, 310, 314; adolescent patients at, 248-9, 293-4; affiliated with Albert Einstein College of Medicine, 246; anesthesiology at, 218, 222, 227, 247; Asklepitron at, 223; Blood Bank at, 295; Board of Trustees of, 244, 252-3, 254, 297, 303, 304-7; budget deficits of, 229, 267; and budget growth curve, 252; Cardiac Catheterization Laboratory at, 290; cardiac patients at, 289, 296; Cardiothoracic Service at, 289; Cardiovascular Group at, 216; clinical chiefships established by, 226; Clinical Research Center established by, 247; Clinical Sciences Department at, new, 292; and Community Advisory Board, 260, 261, 297; construction programs of, 250, 303; coronary bypass surgery at, 290-1; Cranio-Facial Center at, 266; Day Care Center opened by, 215; dermatology at, 222, 258, 295; Diagnostic Radiology Division at, 222, 223; Dialysis Unit at, 254; divisions of Medicine at, 222, 295; elderly patients at, 309, 310; Emergency Medical Services at, 295; endocrinology at, 258, 295; ethical issues within, 273; expenditures of (1966-76), 251-2, 267; Family Medicine Department at, 257; and full-time principle in medicine, 297, 298; gastroenterology at, 222, 243, 258, 295; geriatrics at, 309-10; Headache Unit at, 267; hematology at, 222, 257, 258, 266, 295; immuno-hematology at, 258, 295; income of (1971), 267; Intensive Care Unit at, 255; Kidney Service at, 254; kidney transplants at, 254, 255; Medicine Department at, 222, 256-7, 294, 295; microsurgery at, 288; and Morrisania Hospital, involvement with, 235-6; Neoplastic Diseases Division at, 222, 247; neurology at, 222, 227, 267, 297; non-salaried

Index

Index